GET
THROUGH

MRCS
Anatomy

This book is dedicated to Zachary

GET THROUGH

MRCS
Anatomy

Second edition

Simon Overstall MBBS MRCS FRACS (Plas)
Consultant Plastic Surgeon, Royal Melbourne Hospital,
Melbourne, Australia

Amit Zaveri MBBS (Lon) BSc (Hons) MRCS
Orthopaedic Research Fellow, King's College Hospital,
London, UK

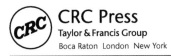

CRC Press
Taylor & Francis Group
Boca Raton London New York

CRC Press is an imprint of the
Taylor & Francis Group, an **informa** business

First published in Great Britain in 2006 by the Royal Society of Medicine Press
This second edition published in 2012 by
Hodder Arnold, an imprint of Hodder Education, a division of Hachette UK

338 Euston Road, London NW1 3BH

http://www.hodderarnold.com

British Library Cataloguing in Publication Data
A catalogue record for this book is available from the British Library

Library of Congress Cataloging-in-Publication Data
A catalog record for this book is available from the Library of Congress

ISBN-13   978-1-4441-7019-1

1 2 3 4 5 6 7 8 9 10

Development Editor: Sarah Penny
Project Editor: Stephen Clausard
Production Controller: Joanna Walker
Cover Design: Helen Townson

Typeset in Minion-Regular 10pts by Data Page (India) Pvt. Ltd.
Printed and bound in India

What do you think about this book? Or any other Hodder Arnold title?
Please visit our website: www.hodderarnold.com

CONTENTS

Preface   vii
Acknowledgements   viii
Introduction   ix

1 Limbs and spine   Questions   1
                            Answers   21
2 Head and neck   Questions   42
                            Answers   54
3 Thorax and abdomen   Questions   72
                            Answers   91
4 Neuroscience   Questions   109
                            Answers   118

The original 'Get through MRCS: Anatomy Vivas' was published some 5 years ago and proved to be a very popular little book. The aim was not to present an exhaustive anatomy text or a list of all the possible questions candidates could be asked, but rather a group of selected questions that were remembered by previous candidates that represented frequently occurring topics. These were presented with model answers and explanations that would both educate the reader and highlight gaps in their knowledge that could be filled by reading the relevant chapter in a good anatomy text.

In 2010 the format of the intercollegiate MRCS exam changed. Instead of the traditional viva voce, a more standardised and structured OSCE style exam is now used to test anatomy. The candidates rotate around 20 stations (including two resting stations), each lasting 10 minutes (including 1 minute of reading time). All stations have an equal value. Anatomy and Surgical Pathology represents one of the four domains. There are three anatomy stations, two generic and one specialty choice. The new-style exam allows the candidate to choose an area of specialisation from the following four categories:

1. limbs and spine
2. head and neck
3. thorax and abdomen
4. neuroscience.

All candidates are expected to have a basic knowledge of all four areas but can select an area for more in-depth questioning. The anatomy stations use a variety of props to prompt questions, including wet specimens, radiological images, photographs, bones and live models. The examiners usually start with pure anatomy questions and then lead on to clinically relevant points, operative details and surgical pathology, all around the same topic. There will be a variety of questions ranging in difficulty, usually starting easier and progressing to greater depth if answered well.

This second edition has been designed to match the new format of the exam and to add new questions that have been asked recently. As with the original book we have presented a selection of questions from across the regions with answers and explanations.

ACKNOWLEDGEMENTS

Many thanks again to Dr Norman Eisenberg and Dr Chris Briggs (Anatomedia) at the University of Melbourne and Dr Gerry Ahern and the 'Dartos Contractors' of Monash University for the use of the anatomical images in this second edition.

INTRODUCTION

Anatomy is one of the toughest subjects for medical students and surgical trainees. It requires a good memory for details and the ability to think in three dimensions. There is, unfortunately, no shortcut to learning the subject. Read through the books and then consolidate your knowledge using dissected cadavers, plastic or computer models or time spent in the operating theatre. Ask questions whenever you assist in theatre. Most surgeons are only too keen to show off their hard-earned knowledge of anatomy.

Anatomy is more than just rote learning tables, however. You need to understand the basic layout of the body, the concepts of fascia and compartments, and then visualise the three-dimensional model in your mind's eye. There are a few simple rules that may help you deduce many surprise viva questions.

Some people find mnemonics a useful way to learn anatomy. My advice would be to use mnemonics only in conjunction with an understanding and a mental picture of the region. It is very easy to remember the mnemonic but to forget what the dirty rhyme or acronym actually stands for. I have included some of the cleaner mnemonics for those of you who haven't heard them before.

The best time to use this book is in the weeks running up to the exam, having already read through a good anatomy textbook and atlas. Close your textbooks and then ask yourself the questions in this book. Better still, find someone else to ask you the questions. Pretend you are in the exam and try to verbalise the answers in full for each question before checking the answers. You'll be surprised how difficult it is to accurately and concisely explain a topic you thought you knew well. It is much better to practise this technique now before the exam. Don't worry if you can't recite all the answers as listed in this book – these are designed as model answers. You won't fail for missing some of the finer details.

This book is designed to highlight gaps in your knowledge. Go and read the relevant chapter in the textbook if you don't feel you answered a particular question well enough.

Here are some general tips that are useful for any viva voce:

1. Ask for the question to be repeated or rephrased if you didn't hear or didn't understand it the first time.
2. Stop and think for a few seconds before shouting out the answer. This gives you a chance to organise your thoughts.
3. Try to present your answer in a clear, logical way. If possible, break down your answer into headings or topics. For example, 'What are the branches of the axillary artery?' 'The axillary artery has three parts relating to the relation of the pectoralis minor muscle. The first part has one branch, the second part has two

branches and the third part has three branches. They are as follows ...' A snappy, concise answer like this will make it clear to the examiner that you know your stuff – he or she will then tick the box and move on to the next question. Dragging out a long-winded list of the branches in a random order will annoy the examiners and lead to lower scores.

4. Always look the examiners in the eye. You will often be handed a bone or other prop to lead the questions. It is a bad idea (but it often happens) to mumble the answer while staring at the object. Look at and speak to the examiners, and use the prop only to demonstrate certain points in your answer.

5. Expect the unexpected. There will always be a question you don't know the answer to. If this happens it is reasonable to make an informed guess – but if you really don't know, say so. The examiners will move on to another topic (ideally one that you do know) and you'll have another chance to pick up points.

6. Put the bad questions behind you. Don't dwell on the question you didn't know or answered badly. Try not to get too flustered. When a question has finished, move on and concentrate on the next subject.

7. When shown a cadaver or wet specimen, take time to orient yourself. Find a point of reference that you recognise and work your way round from this. For example, if you're shown the brachial plexus, look for the 'M' shape that is formed by the confluence of the branches from the medial and lateral cords that form the median nerve. You should then be able to work your way back from this landmark and deduce the rest.

8. Be concise with your answers. Avoid waffling if you can answer the question in a few clear sentences. This will impress the examiners and allow you more time to gain points in the next question.

Question 1

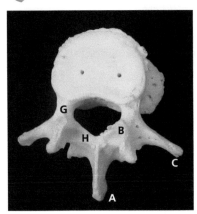 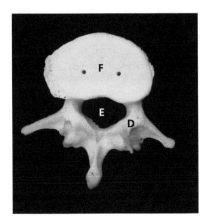

1. From which part of the spinal column is this vertebra?
2. What characteristics help you identify its position?
3. From which orientation are the photos taken?
4. Identify the parts labelled A–F.
5. Point out the lamina and the pedicle using the markers G and H.
6. What are the articulations between adjacent vertebrae?
7. What type of joints are these?
8. What pathological phenomena commonly affect these joints?
9. Which ligaments support the vertebral bodies?
10. Identify the location of the ligamentum flavum.
11. What is the composition of an intervertebral disc?
12. Describe the pathology involved in intervertebral disc prolapse.
13. What is the most common pattern of intervertebral disc herniation?
14. Which are the most commonly affected nerve roots?
15. What is the content of the nucleus pulposus?

Question 2

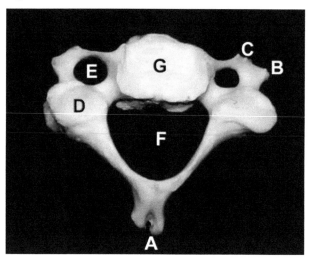

1. What is this specimen?
2. What characteristics help you identify it?
3. Identify the parts labelled A–G.
4. Describe the articulations between such adjacent vertebrae.
5. What is the uncus, and what is its significance?
6. What travels through the transverse foramen?
7. What attachments are given by the anterior and posterior tubercles?
8. What is the significance of the spinous process of C7?
9. Summarise the ligamentous anatomy of the cervical spine.
10. What is a cervical rib?
11. What is the clinical significance of a cervical rib?

Question 3

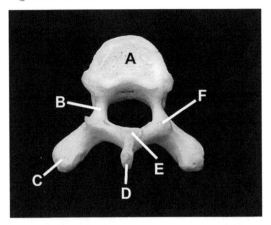

1. From what region of the spine is this vertebra?
2. What features help you identify its position?
3. Identify the parts labelled A–F.
4. How many spinal nerves are there?
5. Describe the articulations between ribs and thoracic vertebrae.
6. What landmarks are used when performing a lumbar puncture?
7. Through which layers does the needle pass during a lumbar puncture?
8. Describe the anatomy of the sympathetic chain.

Question 4

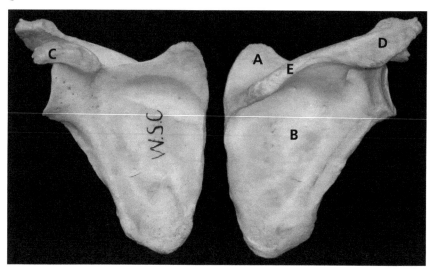

1. Identify the bony specimen. From which side is it?
2. Identify the points labelled A–E.
3. Which muscles comprise the shoulder rotator cuff?
4. Describe the muscles and movements involved in raising the arm above the head.
5. What is the cause of the 'painful arc'?
6. What is the brachial plexus?
7. What are the five regions of the brachial plexus called?
8. Describe the origins of the brachial plexus.
9. How many branches are there from the divisions of the brachial plexus?
10. Draw a simple line diagram of the brachial plexus, and label the branches.
11. What muscles do the branches of the posterior cord of the brachial plexus supply?
12. What muscle is supplied by the long thoracic nerve, and how may you test it?

Question 5

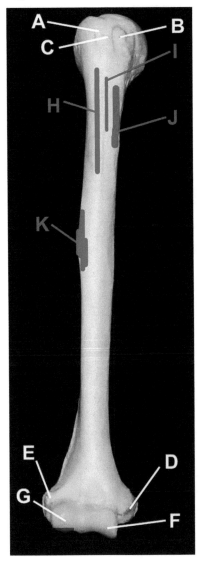

1. Identify this bone.
2. Identify the bony prominences labelled A–G.
3. Which muscles attach to the points marked H–K?
4. What are the boundaries of the axilla?
5. What are the contents of the axilla?
6. Name the branches of the axillary artery.
7. What is the clavipectoral fascia?
8. What structures pierce it?
9. What is the quadrangular space, and what structures pass through it?
10. Which nerves can be damaged by fracture of the humerus?

Question 6

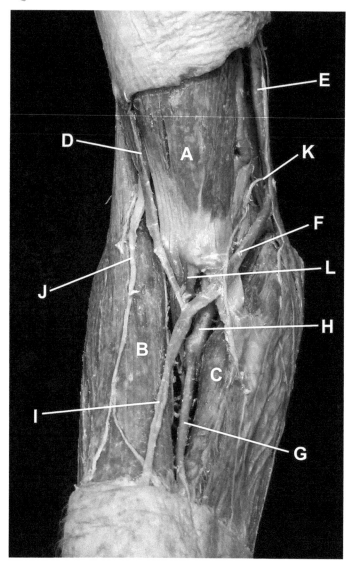

1. What is the anatomical region in the specimen?
2. Identify the muscles A–C.
3. Identify the other structures D–L.
4. What are the boundaries of the cubital fossa?
5. What forms the floor of the cubital fossa?
6. Which structures make up its roof?
7. What are the contents of the cubital fossa?
8. Where does the median cubital vein lie relative to the bicipital aponeurosis?
9. Describe the anatomy of the cubital tunnel.
10. What is the clinical significance of the cubital tunnel?

Question 7

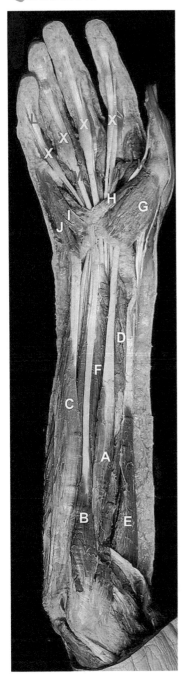

1. Identify the muscles labelled A–J.
2. Identify the tendons labelled K–M.
3. What happens to the tendons at the points marked X?

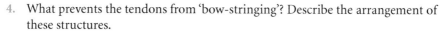

4. What prevents the tendons from 'bow-stringing'? Describe the arrangement of these structures.
5. From where does the musculocutaneous nerve arise?
6. What muscles does it supply?
7. Does this nerve have a sensory component?
8. Describe the arrangement of the muscles in the flexor compartment of the forearm.
9. What is the nerve supply to the forearm flexor compartment muscles?
10. What are the actions of the flexor digitorum profundus and flexor digitorum superficialis muscles? How would you test these muscles?
11. Which superficial flexor muscle is congenitally absent in around 10% of the population? What is the clinical significance of this?

Question 8

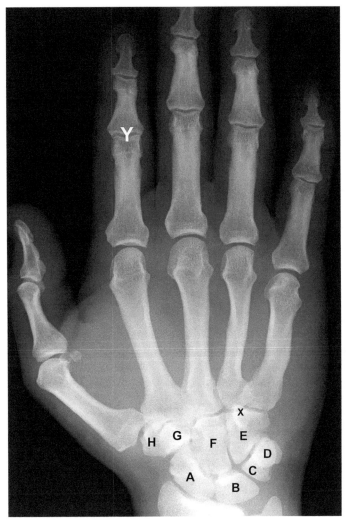

1. Name the carpal bones labelled A–H.
2. What is marked by point X?
3. What joint is marked by point Y?
4. Which of the carpal bones provide attachment for the flexor retinaculum?
5. How many compartments are there in the extensor retinaculum, and what runs through each one?
6. Which structures pass through the carpal tunnel?
7. Which structures are cut through during open carpal tunnel release procedure? Which structures are at risk of damage?
8. What is the yellow-shaded area on the dorsum of the hand known as?

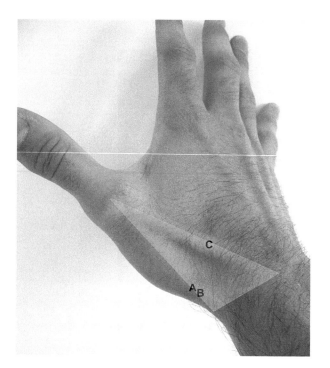

9. What are the boundaries of this region? Which tendons are labelled A–C?
10. What are the contents of this anatomical region?
11. A fracture of which bone may present as tenderness in this region?
12. What is a complication of a fracture of this bone? Describe the pathological process responsible.

Question 9

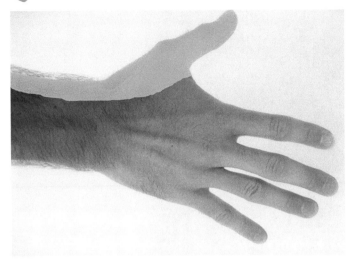

1. Which dermatome is highlighted by the yellow-shaded area?
2. What is the motor supply to the hand?
3. Name the three hypothenar muscles.
4. What is the function of the interossei?
5. What do the lumbricals do?
6. What are the terminal branches of the radial artery in the hand?
7. What is the clinical name for pathological enlargement of the proximal interphalangeal joints and distal interphalangeal joints of the hand?
8. Which tendons of the fingers are contained within a sheath? What is the clinical significance of this?
9. Describe the pathological process that commonly affects the palmar fascia.

Question 10

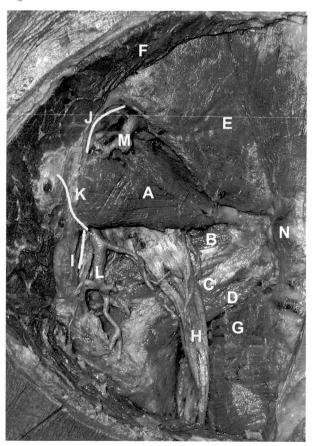

1. This is the posterior aspect of the gluteal region. From which side is it?
2. Identify the muscles labelled A–G.
3. What nerve exits the pelvis above muscle A?
4. What muscle does this nerve supply?
5. What is the function of these muscles?
6. How would damage to this nerve manifest itself?
7. Identify the nerves H–K.
8. Identify the arteries L and M.
9. From which artery do these two vessels originate?
10. Through which foramen do these two arteries exit the pelvis?
11. What bony prominence is marked by N, and which muscles insert here?
12. What structures are cut through during the posterior approach to the hip joint?
13. What nerves are at risk during this approach?

Question 11

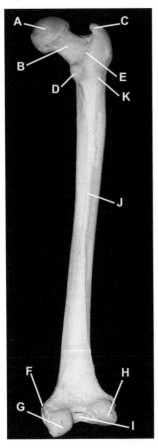

1. What is this bone, and from which side is it?
2. Identify the parts labelled A–K.
3. Describe the blood supply to the head and neck of the femur.
4. What is the significance of this?
5. Name the muscles in the anterior compartment of the thigh.
6. What is the nerve to the medial compartment of the thigh?
7. What cutaneous nerve supplies sensation to the outside of the thigh?
8. What dermatome is this?
9. What are the surface markings of this nerve (as used to perform a nerve block)?
10. What are the nerve roots of the sciatic nerve?
11. What are the terminal branches of the sciatic nerve?
12. How would you test the sensory and motor function of the L5 nerve root.

Question 12

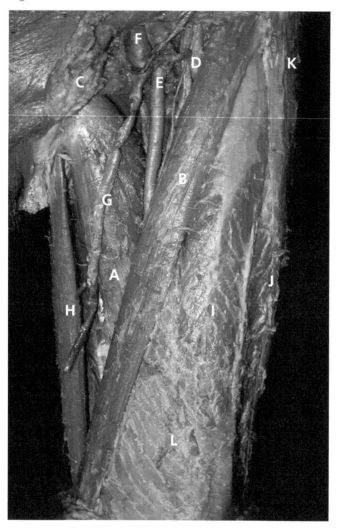

1. What are the boundaries of the femoral triangle? Identify these structures using the labels on the specimen.
2. What are the contents of the femoral triangle?
3. Identify the structures labelled A–L.
4. What structures form the floor of the femoral triangle?
5. What makes up its roof?
6. Describe the surface markings of the femoral artery.
7. What is the femoral sheath?
8. With which anterior abdominal layer is the femoral sheath in continuity?
9. What is the femoral canal?
10. What is the femoral ring, and what are its boundaries?
11. What is its significance to the surgeon?

Question 13

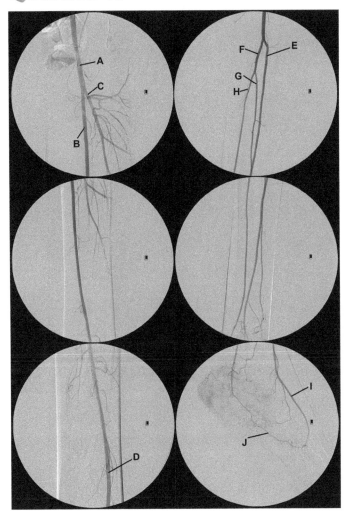

1. What investigation is this?
2. Describe the vascular supply to the leg using the images above.
3. Identify the vessels labelled A–J.
4. Describe the course of the long saphenous vein.
5. What nerve runs in close proximity to the long saphenous vein?
6. Where does this nerve arise?
7. What does this nerve supply?
8. What is the relevance of this to the vascular surgeon?
9. What is the subsartorial (Hunter's) canal?
10. What are its boundaries?
11. Which structures run through it?
12. What is the clinical significance of this canal?

Question 14

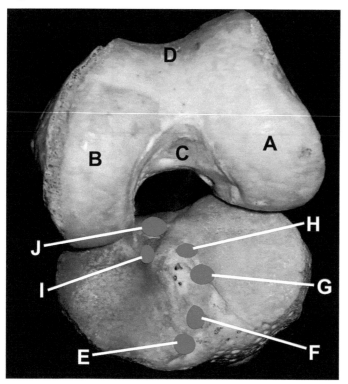

1. What joint is this, and from what side of the body is it?
2. What are the names of the points A–D?
3. What attaches to points E–J?
4. What sort of bone is the patella?
5. What is the function of the patella?
6. Describe the normal position of the lateral collateral ligament.
7. What is the function of the cruciate ligaments?
8. Which of the cruciates is the strongest?
9. How would you test the cruciate ligaments clinically?
10. What is the 'unhappy triad' of knee injuries?

Question 15

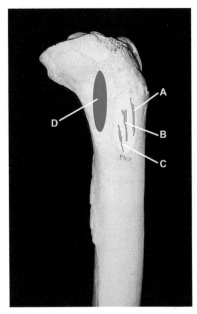

1. What bone is this?
2. What is the name of the area shaded in yellow?
3. What attaches here to points A–C?
4. What is the innervation of these muscles?
5. What attaches to point D?
6. Where does the patellar ligament attach?
7. What is the clinical significance of the yellow-shaded area?

Question 16

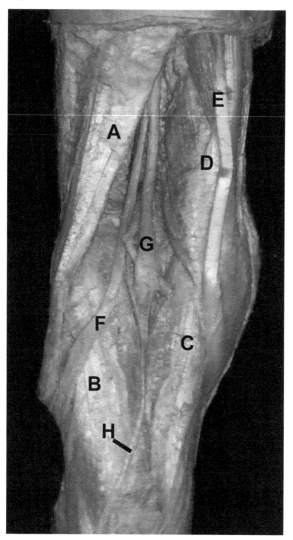

1. Identify the structures labelled A–H.
2. What does structure F divide into?
3. What are the boundaries of the popliteal fossa?
4. What structures are contained within the popliteal fossa?
5. Where does the popliteal artery begin?
6. At what level does the popliteal artery bifurcate?
7. Into which two vessels does the popliteal artery branch?
8. What is the action of the popliteus muscle?
9. What is a Baker's cyst?

Question 17

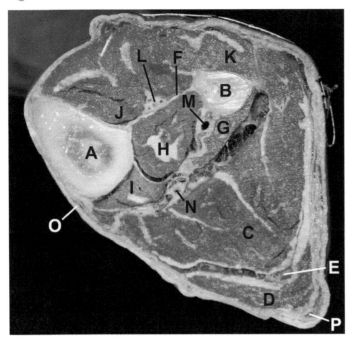

1. How many compartments are there in the leg?
2. What are the structures labelled A–K?
3. Identify the arteries labelled L–N.
4. What are the names of the superficial structures labelled O and P?
5. What nerves run next to the structures labelled O and P?
6. What nerves run next to the arteries labelled L and N?
7. What muscles lie in the anterior compartment?
8. Describe the course of the common peroneal nerve in the leg.
9. What is the clinical significance of the location of the common peroneal nerve?
10. What is the clinical effect of damage to this nerve?
11. What is lower limb compartment syndrome?

Question 18

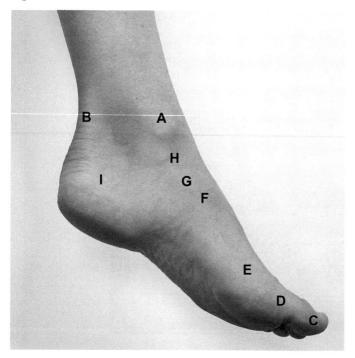

1. What is the name of the bony prominence labelled A?
2. What structures pass behind (posterior to) this landmark?
3. What is the name of the structure palpable at point B?
4. Which muscles contribute to this structure?
5. What are the nerve supplies to these muscles?
6. Which bones can be palpated at points C–I?
7. What is the sustentaculum tali?
8. Where would you palpate the foot pulses?
9. What is the sensory nerve supply to the dorsal first web space of the foot?
10. Describe the muscle layers of the sole of the foot.
11. What other structures run in these layers?
12. What is plantar fasciitis?

LIMBS AND SPINE –
ANSWERS

Question 1 – Answers

1. This is a vertebra from the lumbar region of the spinal column.
2. Lumbar vertebrae have the following characteristics:
   - large kidney-shaped body
   - small vertebral canal
   - massive transverse and spinous processes (not sloping)
   - large pedicles.
3. The photograph on the left is the superior view and the photograph on the right is the inferior view.
4. A – spinous process
   B – inferior articular process and facet
   C – transverse process
   D – superior articular facet
   E – vertebral foramen
   F – vertebral body.
5. G is the pedicle (between the body and arch) and H is the lamina (between the transverse and spinous process).
6. The vertebral arches articulate one with another by superior and inferior articular facets bilaterally.
7. These facet joints are synovial in type. They are oriented in the sagittal plane and allow limited flexion, extension and lateral flexion, but they do not permit rotation.
8. The facet joints in the lumbar region are commonly affected by the degenerative pathological process of osteoarthritis.
9. The vertebral bodies are strengthened by the anterior and posterior longitudinal ligaments on their anterior and posterior surfaces, respectively.
10. The ligamentum flavum is located on the posterior boundaries of the intervertebral foramina (against the facet joints), thereby binding together adjacent laminae.
11. The vertebral bodies are joined together by intervertebral discs, which are secondary cartilaginous joints. The periphery of the discs is made of tough fibrous tissue known as the annulus fibrosis. The centre of the disc is not fibrous but is composed of a gelatinous matrix called the nucleus pulposus.
12. In intervertebral disc prolapse, there is degeneration and subsequent weakening of the annulus fibrosis, resulting in the nucleus pulposus herniating through a

split in the posterior surface of the annulus. This can cause compression of the spinal cord or spinal nerve roots, culminating in neurological symptoms.

13. Disc herniation most commonly occurs in an eccentric manner, as opposed to a central pattern, thereby more often causing compression of spinal nerve roots rather than the spinal cord itself.

14. The most commonly affected nerve root levels are L4/L5 and L5/S1.

15. The nucleus pulposus consists of collagenous fibres (type II collagen) in a mucoprotein gel containing polysaccharide.

Question 2 – Answers

1. This is a typical cervical vertebra (C3–C7 are typical cervical vertebrae). This picture happens to be of a C3 vertebra.

2. Characteristics of cervical vertebrae are:
   large, triangular vertebral foramen
   small transverse processes containing a foramen
   small and wide body
   short and bifid (C3–C5) spinous process.

3. A – spinous process
   B – posterior tubercle of transverse process
   C – anterior tubercle of transverse process
   D – superior articular process
   E – transverse foramen
   F – vertebral foramen
   G – body.

4. The vertebral arches articulate with each other by way of synovial joints. These lie almost on the coronal plane in the cervical region, thereby allowing for lateral flexion, forward flexion and extension.

5. The uncus is a small upturned lip on the upper lateral margins of the cervical vertebrae. They form uncovertebral joints with successive vertebrae and allow rotational movements.

6. The right and left vertebral arteries (branches of the subclavian arteries) ascend towards the skull through the lined-up transverse foramina of the cervical vertebrae.

7. The anterior and posterior tubercles give attachments to scalenus anterior, scalenus medius and scalenus posterior muscles in the neck.

8. The spinous process of C7 is the most prominent of the cervical vertebrae and can be easily palpated; it can therefore be used to identify spines of vertebrae below this level. The seventh cervical vertebra is called the vertebra prominens.

9. The vertebral bodies are strengthened by the **anterior and posterior longitudinal ligaments** on their anterior and posterior surfaces, respectively. The vertebral processes are also joined by **supraspinous** and **interspinous ligaments** (between spinous processes) and **intertransverse ligaments** (between transverse processes).

10. A cervical rib is a supernumerary rib that arises from the anterior tubercle of the seventh cervical vertebra as a congenital abnormality.

11. A cervical rib can sometimes cause impingement of nearby anatomical structures, resulting in reduced blood flow in the subclavian vessels (see the question on subclavian steal syndrome, p. 63) or stretching of the lower brachial plexus nerve roots. T1 root impingement can present with weakness of the small muscles of the hand, for example.

Question 3 – Answers

1. This vertebra is from the thoracic region of the spinal column (this is the inferior aspect of T6).
2. The thoracic vertebrae have the following characteristics:
   - heart-shaped body
   - small and circular vertebral foramen
   - long transverse processes that angle posteriorly
   - facets on the sides of the body for articulation with the ribs
   - long spinous processes that angle inferiorly.
3. A – body
   B – pedicle
   C – transverse process (sloping posteriorly)
   D – spinous process (sloping inferiorly)
   E – lamina
   F – inferior articular process.
4. There are 31 pairs of spinal nerves:
   - 8 cervical
   - 12 thoracic
   - 5 lumbar
   - 5 sacral
   - 1 coccygeal.
5. Every thoracic vertebra articulates with a pair of ribs by means of demifacets on the lateral aspects of the bodies (except the first T1, and the last two T11/T12). Each rib articulates with the vertebra at its own level and also with the vertebra above, the head of the rib thereby traversing the intervertebral discs. Additionally, there are further synovial joints between the ribs and transverse processes of vertebrae at their own level. Ribs at T1, T11 and T12 articulate with their own level only.
6. A line drawn between the iliac crests (supracrestal plane) will intersect the vertebral column at the level of L4. A lumbar puncture needle should be inserted into the space between the L4 and L5 vertebrae.
7. The needle will pass through the following layers:
   - skin
   - subcutaneous fat
   - deep fascia
   - supraspinous ligament
   - interspinous ligament
   - ligamentum flavum
   - dura mater
   - arachnoid mater.
   Note: there are no muscles in the midline.

8. The cell bodies of the sympathetic nerve cells lie within the lateral horn of grey matter of the spinal cord from the level of T1 to L2. Preganglionic fibres pass from these cell bodies through the anterior roots of the spinal cord to enter the anterior rami of the spinal nerves of T1 to L2. From here, these fibres pass through white rami communicantes to enter the sympathetic chain, where they synapse with postganglionic fibres. These synapses occur at the level of the nerve root, or the preganglionic fibres may ascend or descend a level. Some fibres pass through the sympathetic chain without synapsing to form splanchnic nerves. The postganglionic fibres then return to the anterior rami via the grey rami communicantes for distribution to the target organs. (The white rami communicantes contain unmyelinated fibres, and the grey rami communicantes contain myelinated fibres.) The sympathetic chain receives white rami communicantes from the T1 to L2 levels only, but the chain extends up and down the entire length of the spinal column. There are three cervical ganglia: superior, middle and inferior. Usually the inferior cervical ganglion is fused with the first thoracic ganglion to form the larger stellate ganglion, which lies just above the neck of the first rib.

Question 4 – Answers

1. This is the right scapula. The image on the left is the ventral view, and the image on the right is the dorsal view.
2. A – supraspinous fossa
    B – infraspinous fossa
    C – coracoid process
    D – acromion
    E – spine of scapula.
3. The rotator cuff is made up of four muscles (remember 'SITS'):
    - supraspinatus
    - infraspinatus
    - teres minor
    - subscapularis.
    These four muscles blend their tendinous insertions into the articular capsule of the glenohumeral joint. This arrangement holds the humerus tightly in position, giving greater stability to the shoulder joint but still allowing a large range of movement.
4. Many types of movement occur at the shoulder joint, including flexion, extension, abduction, adduction, circumduction and rotation. In **forward flexion**, there is contraction of the **anterior fibres of the deltoid**. During **abduction**, **supraspinatus** initiates the movement, which is subsequently taken over by the **deltoid**. Beyond 90° abduction the humerus is rotated laterally by **subscapularis, teres major** and **infraspinatus**. In addition, there is rotation of the scapula to elevate the glenoid, as produced by the **trapezius** and **serratus anterior**.
5. The 'painful arc' is caused by disorders of the rotator cuff muscle tendons, most commonly that of supraspinatus. Inflammation of this tendon and of the

overlying subacromial bursa due to degeneration or trauma results in painful abduction of the arm between 60° and 120°.

6. The brachial plexus is a large network of nerves that originates in the neck and extends into the axilla, giving rise to most of the nerves that supply the upper limb.

7. The brachial plexus is divided into five regions:
   - roots
   - trunks
   - divisions
   - cords
   - branches.

8. The brachial plexus originates from the ventral primary rami of C5, C6, C7, C8 and T1.

9. None: all the branches exit the brachial plexus before or after the divisions.

10. Practise drawing the basic pattern of the brachial plexus using a simplified line diagram like the one shown here. Then fill in the branches:

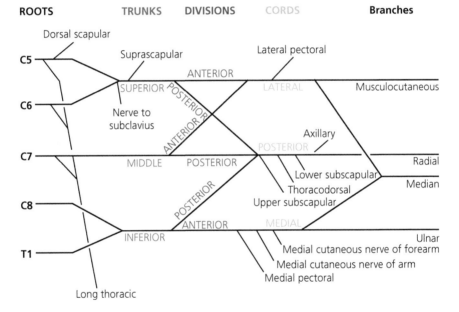

- **Three branches from the roots:**
  - dorsal scapular nerve from C5
  - nerve to subclavius from C5 and C6
  - long thoracic nerve from C5 and C6 and C7.
- **One branch from the upper trunk:**
  - suprascapular nerve.
- **Three branches from the lateral cord:**
  - lateral pectoral nerve
  - lateral root of median nerve
  - musculocutaneous nerve.
- **Five branches from the posterior cord:**
  - upper subscapular nerve

    – thoracodorsal nerve

    – lower subscapular nerve

    – axillary nerve

    – radial nerve.

  Five branches from the medial cord:

    – medial pectoral nerve

    – medial cutaneous nerve of arm

    – medial cutaneous nerve of forearm

    – medial root of median nerve

    – ulnar nerve.

11. The posterior cord of the brachial plexus supplies the muscles that form the posterior border of the axilla, the deltoid and the posterior muscles of the arm and forearm. The branches are as follows:

    upper subscapular nerve – subscapularis

    thoracodorsal nerve – latissimus dorsi

    lower subscapular nerve – subscapularis and teres major

    axillary nerve – deltoid, teres minor

    radial nerve – triceps, all the extensor muscles of the forearm.

12. Serratus anterior is supplied by the long thoracic nerve (of Bell) (– C567 bells in heaven). To test this muscle you should ask the patient to face a wall and push both hands forward against it. Weakness of serratus anterior will cause characteristic winging of the scapula on that side.

Question 5 – Answers

1. This is a right humerus. (With the humeral head pointing inwards, the capitulum and trochlea point forwards.)

2. A – greater tubercle

    B – lesser tubercle

    C – intertubercular (bicipital) groove

    D – medial epicondyle

    E – lateral epicondyle

    F – trochlea

    G – capitulum.

3. H – pectoralis major

    I – latissimus dorsi

    J – teres major ('lady between two majors')

    K – deltoid.

4. The axilla is a pyramidal intermuscular space. Its boundaries are as follows:

    apex – cervicoaxillary canal (convergence of clavicle, scapula and first rib)

    anterior – pectoralis major and minor muscles

    base – axillary fascia

    posterior – subscapularis, teres major, latissimus dorsi muscles (superior to inferior)

- **medial** – upper three ribs, intercostal spaces and serratus anterior muscle
- **lateral** – intertubercular groove of humerus, short head of biceps, coracobrachialis tendon.

5. The contents of the axilla are:
   - axillary artery and its branches
   - axillary vein and its tributaries
   - axillary lymph nodes:
     – level 1 (below pectoralis minor)
     – level 2 (behind pectoralis minor)
     – level 3 (above pectoralis minor)
   - brachial plexus – cords and branches
   - fat.

6. The axillary artery is divided into three parts. The **first part** is medial to pectoralis minor and has one branch:
   - superior thoracic artery.

   The **second part** is behind pectoralis minor and has two branches:
   - thoracoacromial trunk
   - lateral thoracic artery.

   The **third part** is lateral to pectoralis minor and has three branches:
   - subscapular artery
   - anterior circumflex humeral artery
   - posterior circumflex humeral artery.

7. The clavipectoral fascia is a thin layer of fibrous tissue that surrounds the pectoralis minor muscle. It attaches superiorly to the clavicle and inferiorly to the axillary fascia. It is thus the suspensory ligament of the axilla below the pectoralis minor.

8. Four structures pierce the clavipectoral fascia. **Two structures pass in:**
   - cephalic vein
   - lymphatic vessels.

   Two structures pass out:
   - lateral pectoral nerve
   - thoracoacromial trunk.

9. The quadrangular space is formed:
   - laterally by the humerus
   - medially by the long head of triceps
   - superiorly by teres minor
   - inferiorly by teres major.

   Passing through this space is the axillary nerve and the posterior circumflex humeral artery.

10. The following nerves may be damaged by fractures of the humerus:
    - the axillary nerve as it passes close to the neck of the humerus in the quadrangular space
    - the radial nerve as it winds around the shaft of the humerus at the junction between the proximal two-thirds and distal third
    - the ulnar nerve as it passes behind the medial epicondyle
    - the median nerve in a supracondylar fracture.

Question 6 – Answers

1. This is the right cubital fossa, a hollow area on the anterior surface of the elbow.
2. A – biceps brachii
   B – brachioradialis
   C – pronator teres.
3. D – cephalic vein
   E – basilic vein
   F – median cubital vein
   G – radial artery
   H – brachial artery
   I – cephalic vein
   J – lateral cutaneous nerve of forearm (termination of musculocutaneous nerve)
   K – medial cutaneous nerve of forearm (branch of medial cord of brachial plexus)
   L – biceps tendon.
4. The cubital fossa is a triangular intermuscular space bounded:
   superiorly by a line connecting the medial and lateral epicondyles of the humerus
   medially by pronator teres
   laterally by brachioradialis.
5. The floor of the cubital fossa is formed from the brachialis and supinator muscles.
6. The roof of the cubital fossa comprises the bicipital aponeurosis, deep fascia of the forearm and skin.
7. The contents of the cubital fossa from lateral to medial are ('TAN'):
   biceps tendon
   brachial artery (with venae comitantes)
   median nerve.
8. The median cubital vein lies superficial to the bicipital aponeurosis.
9. The cubital tunnel has a roof formed by the aponeurotic expansion of the two heads of flexor carpi ulnaris. This spans in an arcade from the medial epicondyle of the humerus to the olecranon process of the ulna. The floor is formed by the medial collateral ligament of the elbow, expanding from the medial border of the olecranon to the base of the epicondyle.
10. The ulnar nerve passes through the cubital tunnel as it runs behind the medial epicondyle. The ulnar nerve can be compressed within the cubital tunnel. This results in ulnar nerve symptoms and signs within the forearm and hand and is termed cubital tunnel syndrome.

Question 7 – Answers

1. A – flexor carpi radialis
   B – palmaris longus
   C – flexor carpi ulnaris
   D – flexor pollicis longus

E – brachioradialis

F – flexor digitorum superficialis

G – abductor pollicis brevis

H – flexor pollicis brevis

I – flexor digiti minimi

J – abductor digiti minimi.

2. K – flexor pollicis longus

L – flexor digitorum profundus to little finger

M – flexor digitorum superficialis to ring finger.

3. The flexor digitorum superficialis tendon splits to insert into the middle phalanges. The flexor digitorum profundus tendon passes through this split in the flexor digitorum superficialis to insert into the base of the distal phalanges.

4. To prevent the flexor tendons from bow-stringing, there are a series of fascial coverings that anchor the tendon to the bony skeleton, while still allowing the tendons to glide smoothly. At the wrist there is the flexor retinaculum and on the fingers there are the annular (A1–5) and cruciate (C1–3) pulleys:

- the A1 pulley is over the metacarpophalangeal joint
- the A3 pulley is over the proximal interphalangeal joint
- the A5 pulley is over the distal interphalangeal joint
- the A2 pulley is over the proximal phalanx (most important pulley)
- the A4 pulley is over the middle phalanx (second most important pulley)
- the C1 pulley lies between A2 and A3
- the C2 pulley lies between A3 and A4
- the C3 pulley lies between A4 and A5.

From proximal to distal the pulleys are A1, A2, C1, A3, C2, A4, C3, A5.

5. The musculocutaneous nerve is the continuation of the lateral cord of the brachial plexus.

6. The musculocutaneous nerve (the 'BBC nerve') supplies the:

- biceps brachii
- brachialis
- coracobrachialis.

7. Yes, it does – hence the name musculo**cutaneous**. After giving off its motor branches, it crosses the lateral border of the biceps tendon and continues as the lateral cutaneous nerve of the forearm. This supplies sensation to the radial half of the volar forearm and also some of the dorsal surface.

8. The forearm flexor muscles are arranged in two layers. The superficial layer has five muscles arranged like five fingers radiating out from the common flexor origin of the medial epicondyle of the humerus (they all cross the elbow joint). From lateral to medial the muscles are:

- pronator teres
- flexor carpi radialis
- flexor digitorum superficialis
- palmaris longus
- flexor carpi ulnaris.

The deep layer has three muscles, which all originate in the forearm (none crosses the elbow joint):

flexor pollicis longus

flexor digitorum profundus

pronator quadratus.

9. They are all supplied by the median nerve, except for the flexor carpi ulnaris and the ulnar half of the flexor digitorum profundus muscles, which are supplied by the ulnar nerve.

10. The **flexor digitorum profundus tendon** inserts into the base of the distal phalanx of the finger. It can be tested by asking the patient to flex the distal interphalangeal joint of that finger. The **flexor digitorum superficialis tendon** inserts into the base of the middle phalanx of the finger. Flexion at the proximal interphalangeal joint can be by contraction of both the flexor digitorum superficialis and the flexor digitorum profundus; to test the function of the flexor digitorum superficialis muscle alone, the patient's flexor digitorum profundus must be inactivated by holding their other fingers out straight and asking the patient to flex their unrestrained finger at the proximal interphalangeal joint. (Remember 'the superficialis splits in two to allow profundus passing through'.)

11. The palmaris longus is absent in around 10% of the population. This muscle has no real functional significance and can therefore be used as a tendon graft. Before harvesting this tendon graft it is wise to test for its presence while the patient is still awake. Ask the patient to make the V-sign with their index and middle fingers and then slowly flex their wrist. The palmaris longus tendon is visible as a separate line just on the ulnar side of the flexor carpi radialis tendon.

Question 8 – Answers

1. The carpal bones can be divided into proximal and distal rows.
   Proximal row:
   A – scaphoid
   B – lunate
   C – triquetrum
   D – pisiform.
   Distal row:
   E – hamate
   F – capitate
   G – trapezoid
   H – trapezium.

2. X marks the hook of the hamate.

3. Y marks the proximal interphalangeal joint of the index finger.

4. The flexor retinaculum attaches to the:
   hook of the hamate and the pisiform on the ulnar aspect
   lateral ridge of trapezium and the tubercle of the scaphoid on the radial aspect.

5. There are six compartments in the extensor retinaculum. From radial to ulnar:
   extensor pollicis brevis and abductor pollicis longus
   extensor carpi radialis longus and extensor carpi radialis brevis
   extensor pollicis longus
   extensor indicis proprius and extensor digitorum communis

- extensor digiti minimi
- extensor carpi ulnaris.

6. The following structures pass through the carpal tunnel:
    - median nerve
    - flexor pollicis longus tendon
    - flexor digitorum profundus tendons (four of them)
    - flexor digitorum superficialis tendons (four of them).

7. During open carpal tunnel decompression the following layers are cut:
    - skin
    - subcutaneous fat
    - palmar fascia
    - (palmaris brevis muscle)
    - flexor retinaculum.

    It is important to divide the entire length of the flexor retinaculum.
    At risk of damage in open carpal tunnel release are:
    - palmar cutaneous branch of the median nerve (sensation to the thenar eminence)
    - recurrent branch of the median nerve (motor branch to thenar muscles)
    - ulnar nerve as it passes through the flexor retinaculum (with an incision too far to the ulnar side of the hand)
    - median nerve
    - superficial palmar arch
    - flexor tendons passing through the carpal tunnel.

8. This area is known as the anatomical snuffbox.

9. The anatomical snuffbox is bounded on the radial side by the abductor pollicis longus (A) and extensor pollicis brevis (B) tendons. On the ulnar side is the extensor pollicis longus (C) tendon. The floor is the scaphoid and trapezium.

10. The contents of the anatomical snuffbox are the radial artery, radial nerve, and extensor carpi radialis longus and brevis tendons.

11. Tenderness in the region of the anatomical snuffbox, particularly after trauma, is suggestive of fracture of the scaphoid.

12. The scaphoid may undergo avascular necrosis of its proximal pole following fractures through the waist. This is because the blood supply of this bone is relatively poor, being mainly into the distal portion via radial artery branches. A fracture through the waist of the scaphoid disrupts this blood supply, leading to anoxic bone death, with subsequent bone loss and collapse. This may present many months after the original trauma with pain and stiffness in the wrist. If left untreated this may progress to disruption of the neighbouring carpal attachments – the 'SNAC wrist' (scaphoid non-union advanced collapse). Early detection of scaphoid fractures and immobilisation in a cast or open reduction and internal fixation will reduce the risk of this complication.

Question 9 – Answers

1. This is the C6 dermatome.

2. All of the intrinsic muscles of the hand are supplied by the ulnar nerve, except for the lateral two lumbricals, opponens pollicis, abductor pollicis brevis and flexor pollicis brevis ('LOAF muscles'), which are supplied by the median nerve.

3. The hypothenar muscles are:
   - abductor digiti minimi
   - flexor digiti minimi brevis
   - opponens digit minimi.
4. There are four dorsal interossei (between the bones) that attach proximally to adjacent sides of the two metacarpals they lie between (i.e. the fourth dorsal interosseous attaches to the fourth and fifth metacarpals) and insert distally on to the base of the proximal phalanx and extensor expansion. The dorsal interossei **ab**duct the fingers. The little finger has a separate abductor (abductor digiti minimi). There are three palmar interossei that attach proximally to the palmar aspect of the second, fourth and fifth metacarpals and insert distally into the base of the proximal phalanx and extensor expansion of the corresponding digit. The palmar interossei **ad**duct the fingers. (Remember 'PAD DAB'.)
5. There are four lumbricals in each hand. They attach proximally to the flexor digitorum profundus tendon, cross the radial side of the corresponding metacarpophalangeal joint, and insert into the extensor expansion of that digit. They flex the metacarpophalangeal joint and extend the interphalangeal joints.
6. The radial artery divides into the princeps pollicis and radialis indicis, and forms the radial side of the deep palmar arch of the hand.
7. Pathological enlargement of the proximal interphalangeal joints gives rise to Bouchard's nodes (characteristic in rheumatoid arthritis). Enlargement of the distal interphalangeal joints is known as Heberden's nodes (characteristic in osteoarthritis).
8. The flexor tendons are contained within synovial sheaths in the hand, whereas the extensor tendons are not. These sheaths extend from the A1 pulley in the palm to the A5 pulley at the distal interphalangeal joint of the fingers. The membranous layer of the flexor sheath for the thumb and little finger often extends further proximally into the wrist to form the radial and ulnar bursae. Infection within the flexor sheath (flexor tenosynovitis) can be severe and necessitates urgent surgical drainage and washout. Infections here can be so devastating for two reasons. First, the rigid fibro-osseous tunnel of the flexor sheath cannot expand in the presence of pus. This leads to raised pressure and subsequent interruption of the blood supply to the flexor tendons. The late sequelae are atrophic tendon ruptures. Second, the resultant scarring within the flexor sheath following infection leads to adhesions between the tendons and the sheath. This leads to reduced tendon excursion, stiffness and loss of function.
9. The palmar aponeurosis seems to be susceptible to progressive hyperplasia and fibrosis, with subsequent thickening and shortening. This leads to a flexion deformity of one or more of the digits, with associated loss of function. This condition is known as Dupuytren's contracture.

Question 10 – Answers

1. This is a photograph of the right gluteal region. (Note: When you are shown a photograph or specimen of the gluteal region, use the piriformis muscle as a landmark to orient yourself.)

2. A – piriformis
   B – superior gemellus
   C – obturator internus
   D – inferior gemellus
   E – gluteus medius
   F – gluteus maximus
   G – quadratus femoris.
3. The superior gluteal nerve exits above the piriformis.
4. The superior gluteal nerve supplies the gluteus medius and gluteus minimus muscles.
5. Gluteus medius and gluteus minimus are abductors of the hip joint.
6. When one foot is raised off the ground during walking, the contralateral gluteus medius and minimus muscles normally contract and act to stabilise and maintain the pelvis in the horizontal plane. Damage to the superior gluteal nerve would cause the patient to have a Trendelenburg gait, whereby dysfunction of the gluteus medius and minimus results in the pelvis falling when the leg is raised.
7. H – sciatic nerve
   I – pudendal nerve
   J – superior gluteal nerve
   K – inferior gluteal nerve.
8. L – inferior gluteal artery
   M – superior gluteal artery.
9. The superior and inferior gluteal arteries are branches of the internal iliac artery.
10. The superior and inferior gluteal arteries exit the pelvis through the greater sciatic foramen.
11. N marks the greater trochanter of the femur. This is the insertion of gluteus medius and minimus, piriformis, superior and inferior gemelli and obturator internus.
12. The following structures are cut through during the posterior approach to the hip joint:
    - skin
    - subcutaneous fat
    - gluteal fascia
    - gluteus maximus
    - the short external rotator muscles
    - hip joint capsule.
13. The sciatic nerve and superior gluteal nerve are at risk during the posterior approach to the hip joint.

Question 11 – Answers

1. This is the posterior aspect of a right femur.
2. A – head of femur
   B – neck of femur

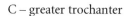

C – greater trochanter

D – lesser trochanter

E – intertrochanteric crest

F – adductor tubercle

G – medial condyle

H – lateral condyle

I – intercondylar fossa

J – linea aspera

K – gluteal tuberosity.

3. The femoral head receives a small amount of blood from the artery within the **ligamentum teres**, but this is usually inadequate alone. The majority of the blood supply comes from the extracapsular arterial ring that lies around the base of the femoral neck. This anastomosis receives branches from the **medial** and **lateral circumflex femoral arteries** and a smaller contribution from the **superior** and **inferior gluteal arteries**. Small vessels from this anastomosis pass through the medulla of the femoral neck to supply the femoral head.

4. Intracapsular fractures of the neck of the femur disrupt the intraosseous blood supply to the femoral head. The blood supply through the ligamentum teres is usually inadequate, thus leading to avascular necrosis of the head of the femur.

5. The anterior thigh muscles are the hip flexors and the knee extensors. They are:

   pectineus

   iliopsoas

   tensor fascia lata

   sartorius

   quadriceps femoris, composed of:

   – rectus femoris

   – vastus lateralis

   – vastus intermedialis

   – vastus medialis.

6. The medial (or adductor) compartment of the thigh is supplied by the obturator nerve.

7. The lateral cutaneous nerve of the thigh supplies sensation to the outside of the thigh.

8. This is the L2 and L3 dermatome.

9. The surface marking of the lateral cutaneous nerve of the thigh is 1–2 cm medial and inferior to the anterior superior iliac spine as the nerve passes below the inguinal ligament.

10. The nerve roots of the sciatic nerve are L3, L4, S1, S2, S3.

11. The terminal branches of the sciatic nerve are the tibial nerve and common peroneal nerve.

12. To clinically examine the L5 nerve root, L5 sensation may be tested at the dorsum of the foot and L5 motor function by testing extensor hallucis longus (lift up big toe).

Question 12 – Answers

1. The boundaries of the femoral triangle are as follows:
   - **medially** – the medial border of adductor longus (A)
   - **laterally** – the medial border of sartorius (B)
   - **superiorly** – the inguinal ligament (C – partially removed in this specimen).
2. The contents of the femoral triangle are, from lateral to medial, the femoral nerve, femoral artery, femoral vein and lymph nodes (remember 'NAVY' – nerve, artery, vein, Y-fronts).
3. A – adductor longus
   B – sartorius
   C – inguinal ligament
   D – femoral nerve
   E – femoral artery
   F – femoral vein
   G – long saphenous vein
   H – gracilis
   I – rectus femoris
   J – vastus lateralis
   K – tensor fascia lata
   L – vastus medialis.
4. The floor of the femoral triangle is formed by the iliacus, psoas tendon, pectineus and adductor longus.
5. The roof of the femoral triangle is formed by the fascia lata.
6. The femoral artery is located 2–3 cm inferior to the midpoint of the inguinal ligament (**not** the mid-inguinal point).
7. The femoral sheath is a fascial tube that extends for 3 cm below the inguinal ligament and surrounds the femoral artery, femoral vein and femoral canal containing lymphatic vessels. It does not contain the femoral nerve.
8. The femoral sheath is a continuation of the extraperitoneal fascia, formed anteriorly by the transversalis fascia and posteriorly by the iliopsoas fascia.
9. The femoral canal is a potential space in the most medial of the compartments of the femoral sheath. It contains fat, lymphatic vessels and Cloquet's node. Superiorly the femoral canal opens into the femoral ring.
10. The femoral ring is the superior mouth of the femoral canal. Its boundaries are:
    - **anterior** – inguinal ligament
    - **posterior** – superior ramus of the pubis covered in the pectineal ligament (of Astley Cooper)
    - **medially** – lacunar ligament
    - **laterally** – fascia around the femoral vein.
11. The femoral ring is where a femoral hernia would occur.

Question 13 – Answers

1. This is a digital subtraction angiogram (DSA) of the left leg.
2. The external iliac artery changes its name to the femoral artery after passing under the inguinal ligament. The femoral (or common femoral) artery gives off a deep branch called the profunda femoris that supplies all the thigh muscles. The continuation of the femoral artery is known by vascular surgeons as the superficial femoral artery. This vessel then becomes the popliteal artery after passing through the adductor hiatus of the adductor magnus tendon. In the popliteal fossa it gives off five genicular branches (superior medial, superior lateral, inferior medial, inferior lateral and middle). The popliteal artery ends by dividing into the anterior tibial artery (smaller) and tibioperoneal trunk (larger). The anterior tibial artery pierces the interosseous membrane and then runs in the anterior compartment of the leg, supplying all the muscles of this compartment. This artery becomes the dorsalis pedis artery after crossing the ankle joint. The tibioperoneal trunk divides into the peroneal artery (larger branch), which runs close to the fibula, and the posterior tibial artery, which runs in the posterior compartment close to the tibial nerve. At the ankle the posterior tibial artery runs behind the medial malleolus and then divides into the medial and lateral plantar arteries. The lateral plantar artery anastomoses with the dorsalis pedis artery at the plantar arch.
3. On the angiogram:
    A – common femoral artery
    B – superficial femoral artery
    C – profunda femoris artery
    D – popliteal artery
    E – anterior tibial artery (note the perpendicular course as it pierces the interosseous membrane)
    F – tibioperoneal trunk
    G – peroneal artery
    H – posterior tibial artery
    I – dorsalis pedis artery
    J – lateral plantar artery.
4. The long saphenous vein starts in the foot as the confluence of the dorsal venous arch and the dorsal vein of the great toe. It passes just anterior to the medial malleolus to climb up the calf, just posterior to the palpable border of the tibia. It passes a hand's breadth behind the medial border of the patella, and continues up the medial aspect of the thigh to then pierce the fascia lata to drain into the femoral vein at the saphenofemoral junction (approximately 2 cm below and lateral to the pubic tubercle). There are numerous perforating veins connecting the deep and superficial venous systems. Some say these are 1 cm below, 1 cm above and 10 cm above the medial malleolus, one in the middle of the calf and one just below the knee. In reality the position of the perforators is quite variable (hence the need for Doppler marking before varicose vein surgery).
5. The saphenous nerve runs close to the long saphenous vein below the knee.
6. The saphenous nerve is a branch of the femoral nerve and passes through the subsartorial canal with the femoral vessels

7. The saphenous nerve supplies sensation to the medial aspect of the calf and foot.
8. The saphenous nerve may be damaged during stripping of the inferior part of the long saphenous vein when treating varicose veins.
9. The subsartorial (adductor or Hunter's) canal is an intermuscular tunnel beneath the middle third of the sartorius muscle. It ends at the adductor hiatus, an opening in the adductor magnus tendon.
10. The boundaries of the subsartorial canal are:
    - **lateral** – vastus medialis
    - **posterior** – adductor longus and adductor magnus
    - **anterior** – sartorius.
11. The contents of the subsartorial canal are the femoral vessels as they pass from the anterior thigh to become the popliteal vessels and two nerves:
    - superficial femoral artery (anterior)
    - femoral vein (posterior)
    - saphenous nerve (note: this nerve does not exit through the adductor hiatus but perforates between gracilis and sartorius to run with the long saphenous vein)
    - nerve to vastus medialis (note: again, this nerve does not exit through the adductor hiatus).
12. The subsartorial canal is an anatomical narrowing and is therefore a common site of turbulent blood flow and atherosclerotic disease.

Question 14 – Answers

1. This is the left knee joint. (Note: The medial condyle or plateau of the tibia is larger than the lateral side. The lateral femoral condyle has a greater prominence on the side of the patella groove to prevent the patella being dislocated laterally with every contraction of the quadriceps – this muscle has a lateral pull.)
2. A – lateral condyle of femur
   B – medial condyle of femur
   C – intercondylar fossa
   D – patella groove.
3. From anterior to posterior, the following structures attach into the tibial plateau:
   E – anterior horn of medial meniscus
   F – anterior cruciate ligament
   G – anterior horn of lateral meniscus
   H – posterior horn of lateral meniscus
   I – posterior horn of medial meniscus
   J – posterior cruciate ligament.
4. The patella is a sesamoid bone (the largest in the body).
5. The function of the patella is to attach the quadriceps tendon to the tibial tuberosity via the patellar ligament, and to increase the power of the quadriceps group by lengthening its leverage.
6. The lateral collateral ligament of the knee runs from the lateral femoral condyle to the head of the fibula.

7. The cruciate ligaments attach the tibia to the femur and are named according to their position of origin on the tibia. The **anterior cruciate ligament** attaches to the anterior part of the intercondylar area of the tibia, just behind the medial meniscus. It runs superiorly and posteriorly to attach into the lateral condyle/intercondylar notch of the femur. It prevents the tibia from being displaced anteriorly from the femur and prevents hyperextension of the knee. The **posterior cruciate ligament** attaches to the posterior aspect of the intercondylar area of the tibia. It runs superiorly and anteriorly to attach into the medial condyle/intercondylar notch of the femur. It prevents the tibia from being displaced posteriorly from the femur and prevents hyperflexion of the knee.
8. The posterior cruciate ligament is stronger than the anterior cruciate ligament.
9. The anterior cruciate ligament is tested by assessing the amount of anterior movement of the tibia relative to the femur with the knee flexed to 90° (anterior drawer test). The posterior cruciate ligament is tested by assessing the amount of posterior movement of the tibia relative to the femur with the knee flexed to 90° (posterior drawer test).
10. The 'unhappy triad' is a combination of rupture of the **anterior cruciate ligament**, rupture of the **medial collateral ligament**, and tear of the **medial meniscus**. It is a serious injury often caused by a direct lateral blow to the knee joint.

Question 15 – Answers

1. This is the medial aspect of the left tibia.
2. This is the pes anserinus (from the Latin for 'goose's foot').
3. Attaching to the pes anserinus is (from anterior to posterior) ('say grace before tea'):
   A – sartorius
   B – gracilis
   C – semitendinosus.
4. The innervation of the pes anserinus muscles is as follows (remember 'SGT FOS'):
   sartorius – femoral nerve
   gracilis – obturator nerve
   semitendinosus – sciatic nerve.
5. The tibial (or medial) collateral ligament attaches to point D.
6. The patellar ligament attaches to the tibial tuberosity.
7. The pes anserinus on the anteromedial tibia is a common site for harvesting the tendons of gracilis and semitendinosus for grafting during anterior cruciate ligament reconstruction surgery.

Question 16 – Answers

1. This is the popliteal fossa (posterior aspect of knee joint):
   A – biceps femoris
   B – lateral head of gastrocnemius
   C – medial head of gastrocnemius
   D – semimembranosus
   E – semitendinosus

F – common peroneal nerve

G – tibial nerve

H – sural nerve.

2. The common peroneal nerve divides into the superficial and deep peroneal nerves.

3. The popliteal fossa is a diamond-shaped intermuscular region on the posterior aspect of the knee. The boundaries are:

    superomedially – semimembranosus and semitendinosus muscles

    inferomedially – medial head of gastrocnemius muscle

    superolaterally – biceps femoris muscle

    inferolaterally – lateral head of gastrocnemius and plantaris muscles

    floor – the capsule of the knee joint, popliteus muscle and femur

    roof – popliteal fascia.

4. The contents of the popliteal fossa are (from deep to superficial):

    popliteal artery

    popliteal vein

    tibial nerve

    common peroneal nerve.

    The popliteal fossa also contains:

    fat

    lymph nodes

    termination of the short saphenous vein as it enters the popliteal vein

    sural nerve

    popliteus bursa

    five genicular branches of the popliteal artery.

5. The popliteal artery is a continuation of the femoral artery. It begins at the adductor hiatus and runs inferolaterally through the popliteal fossa.

6. The popliteal artery bifurcates at the lower border of the popliteus muscle.

7. The popliteal artery branches into the anterior tibial artery and the tibioperoneal trunk.

8. During full extension of the knee joint, there is medial rotation of the femur on the tibia because of the shape of the medial articular surfaces of the femur and tibia. This rotational movement upon full extension has the effect of tensioning all the knee ligaments for maximum stability in this 'locked' position. The popliteus muscle arises from the posterior surface of the tibia and passes superolaterally to insert into the lateral femoral condyle. Its action is to laterally rotate the femur on the tibia at the start of flexion (when from full extension) to unlock the knee joint and permit flexion.

9. A Baker's cyst is a synovial cyst (benign abnormal collection of joint fluid) extruding from the semimembranosus bursa into the popliteal space. It often causes pain as well as being a palpable swelling. Note that this is not a 'true' cyst as there is usually communication with the synovial sac.

Question 17 – Answers

1. There are four compartments in the leg – anterior, lateral, superficial posterior and deep posterior.

2.　A – tibia
　　B – fibula
　　C – soleus
　　D – gastrocnemius
　　E – plantaris tendon
　　F – interosseous membrane
　　G – flexor hallucis longus
　　H – tibialis posterior
　　I – flexor digitorum longus
　　J – tibialis anterior
　　K – peroneus longus.
3.　L – anterior tibial artery
　　M – peroneal artery
　　N – posterior tibial artery.
4.　O – long saphenous vein
　　P – short saphenous vein.
5.　The saphenous nerve runs with the long saphenous vein, while the sural nerve runs with the short saphenous vein.
6.　The deep peroneal nerve runs in the anterior compartment with the anterior tibial artery. The tibial nerve runs in the deep posterior compartment with the posterior tibial artery.
7.　The following muscles lie in the anterior compartment:
　　tibialis anterior
　　extensor digitorum longus
　　extensor hallucis longus
　　peroneus tertius.
8.　The common peroneal nerve is one of the terminal branches of the sciatic nerve. It runs posterior to the head of the fibula between the lateral head of gastrocnemius and the biceps femoris. It then wraps around the lateral aspect of the neck of the fibula underneath the peroneus longus, descends beneath this muscle and divides into the deep and superficial peroneal branches.
9.　The superficial location of the common peroneal nerve as it wraps around the proximal fibula leaves it susceptible to injury from trauma, surgery and even compression by overly tight plaster casts.
10.　Injury to the common peroneal nerve manifests in the patient as a foot-drop.
11.　Lower limb compartment syndrome is a clinical condition in which swelling within the rigid confines of the fascial compartments of the leg leads to compromise to the circulation. This is a limb-threatening pathological process that, if suspected, requires immediate surgical decompression of all the fascial compartments to restore vascularity.

Question 18 – Answers

1.　This is the medial malleolus.
2.　Passing posterior to the medial malleolus, under the flexor retinaculum, are (from anterior to posterior) (remember 'Tom, Dick and very naughty Harry'):

- tibialis posterior tendon
- flexor digitorum tendon
- posterior tibial artery
- venae comitantes of the posterior tibial artery
- tibial nerve
- flexor hallucis longus tendon.

3. This is the tendo calcaneus or Achilles tendon.
4. The three muscles of the superficial posterior compartment of the leg insert into the calcaneus via the Achilles tendon. They are:
   - gastrocnemius (medial and lateral heads)
   - soleus
   - plantaris.
5. All of the superficial posterior compartment muscles are supplied by the tibial nerve.
6. The bones that can be palpated along the medial border of the foot are:
   C – distal phalanx of great toe
   D – proximal phalanx of great toe
   E – first metatarsal
   F – medial cuneiform
   G – navicular
   H – talus
   I – calcaneus.
7. The sustentaculum tali is a shelf-like projection of the calcaneus that provides support for the talus.
8. The dorsalis pedis pulse is palpated on the dorsum of the foot just lateral to the extensor hallucis longus tendon over the cuneiform bones. The posterior tibial pulse is palpable halfway between the posterior border of the medial malleolus and the tendo Achilles.
9. The deep peroneal nerve supplies sensation to the first web space of the foot.
10. Deep to the plantar fascia there are four muscle layers. From superficial to deep they are:
    - abductor hallucis, abductor digiti minimi, flexor digitorum brevis
    - quadratus plantae, lumbricals (×4) (and tendons of flexor digitorum longus and flexor hallucis longus)
    - flexor hallucis brevis, adductor hallucis, flexor digiti minimi
    - plantar interossei (×3), dorsal interossei (×4) (and tendons of tibialis posterior and peroneus longus).
11. The **medial** and **lateral plantar nerves** run between the first and second layers of muscles. The **medial** and **lateral plantar arteries** also run between the first and second layers of muscles. The **deep plantar arch** is between the third and fourth layers.
12. Plantar fasciitis is an inflammatory process of the plantar fascia and a common cause of inferior heel pain. Longstanding cases often demonstrate bony calcaneal osteophytic spurs. The condition is associated with a history of long periods of weight-bearing, such as running.

Question 19

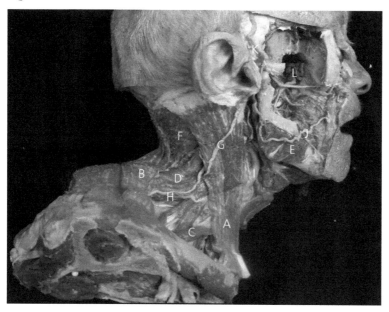

1. Identify the muscles labelled A–F.
2. Identify the nerves labelled G–H.
3. Identify the arteries labelled I–L.
4. Describe the arrangement of the deep fascia of the neck.
5. What are the boundaries of the posterior triangle of the neck?
6. What are the actions of sternocleidomastoid and trapezius?
7. What structures are found in the posterior triangle of the neck?
8. What would be the effect of cutting the spinal accessory nerve in the posterior triangle of the neck?
9. What are the surface markings of the accessory nerve?
10. What are the boundaries of the anterior triangle of the neck?
11. What are the subdivisions of the anterior triangle?
12. What are the boundaries of these triangles?

Question 20

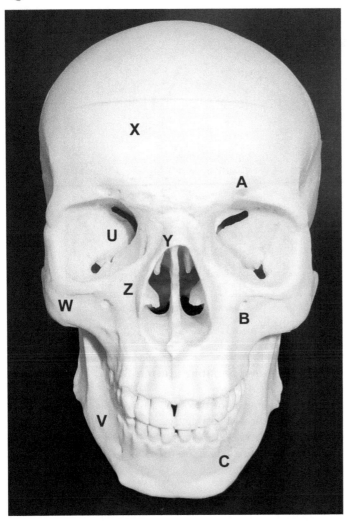

1. What are the names of these foramina (labelled A–C)?
2. What structures pass through them?
3. What are the names of the bones labelled U–Z?
4. What structures run through the superior orbital fissure?
5. Describe the arrangement of the extraocular muscles.
6. What are the actions of the individual extraocular muscles?
7. What is their motor nerve supply?
8. Which bones make up the orbit?
9. What is the clinical appearance of an oculomotor nerve palsy?

Question 21

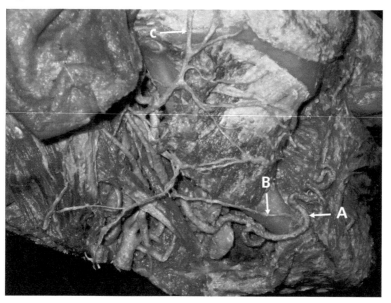

1. Identify the structure labelled A.
2. Where does this originate?
3. Identify the structure labelled B.
4. What are the clinical consequences of cutting structure B?
5. Identify the structure labelled C.
6. What bony structure is C crossing at the tip of the arrow?
7. What are the clinical consequences of cutting C?
8. Describe the path of the facial nerve.
9. What are the branches, and what structures do they supply?
10. How would you quickly test the motor function of the divisions of the facial nerve?
11. What are the surface markings of the parotid gland?
12. What are the surface markings of the parotid (Stenson's) duct?
13. Where does the parotid duct open into the mouth?
14. What nerve runs close to and parallel with the parotid duct?
15. What is the clinical significance of this in a patient with facial trauma?

Question 22

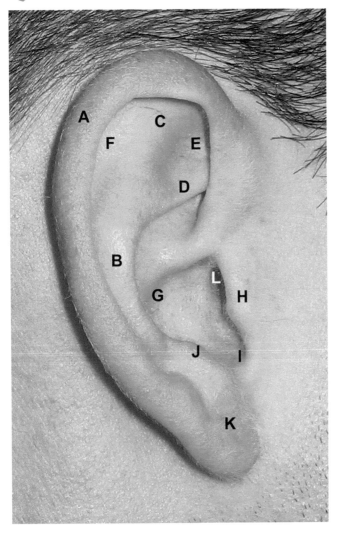

1. Identify the different parts of the ear.
2. What is the sensory nerve supply to the ear?
3. What are the clinical consequences of this pattern of nerve supply?
4. What are the sensory branches of the cervical plexus?
5. Which nerve roots contribute to the cervical plexus?
6. Demonstrate the sensory dermatomes that correspond to the cervical plexus.
7. What is the name of the point where the cervical plexus emerges through the prevertebral fascia?
8. What are the surface markings of this point?
9. Does this point have any clinical uses?

Question 23

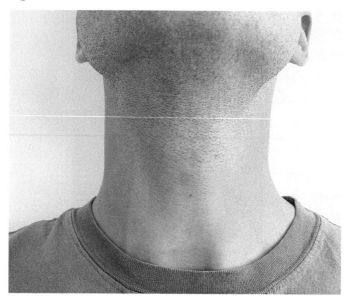

1. Surface mark the following parts of the larynx:
   - hyoid bone
   - thyroid cartilage
   - cricoid cartilage
   - first tracheal ring
   - thyroid membrane
   - laryngeal prominence
   - cricothyroid ligament.
2. List the layers you would cut through during a tracheostomy tube insertion.
3. What are the strap muscles?
4. What are their attachments?
5. What are their actions?
6. What is the motor nerve supply?
7. What is the blood supply to the strap muscles?
8. Why is omohyoid a useful landmark when performing a selective neck dissection?
9. What are the surface markings of the seven cervical vertebrae levels?

Question 24

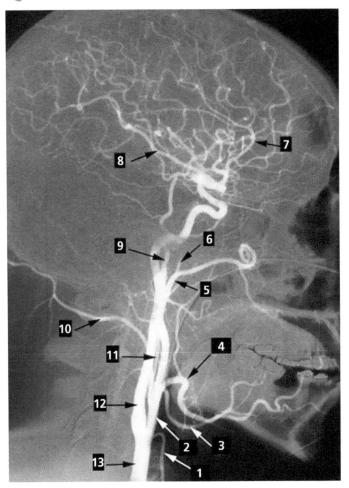

1. Identify the arteries labelled 1–13.
2. List the branches of the external carotid artery.
3. List the branches of the internal carotid artery in the neck.
4. What cervical vertebral level corresponds to the bifurcation of the common carotid artery?
5. What are the branches of the maxillary artery?
6. Which nerves are at risk during surgery to the carotid artery?
7. Where does the vertebral artery originate?
8. Describe the course of this artery as it ascends in the neck.
9. How does the vertebral artery terminate?
10. What is the eponymous name for this anastomosis of arteries?
11. Describe the subclavian steal syndrome.

Question 25

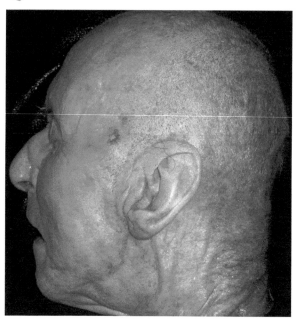

1. What are the layers of the scalp?
2. What is the blood supply to the scalp, and where do these vessels originate?
3. Mark the path of these vessels on the scalp shown.
4. In which layer of the scalp do the blood vessels run?
5. Why do scalp lacerations bleed so profusely?
6. How can this be controlled in the trauma setting?
7. In which layer are flaps raised in the scalp?
8. What is the venous drainage of the scalp?
9. Does this pattern of veins have clinical consequences?
10. Which nerves supply sensation to the scalp?

Question 26

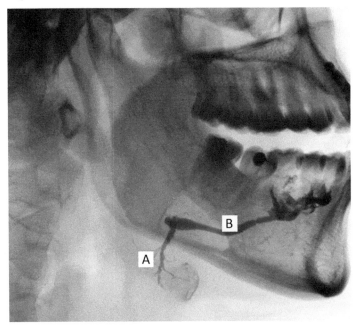

1. What is this investigation?
2. What are the structures labelled A and B?
3. Where is the standard incision made for access to the submandibular gland?
4. Why is it made here?
5. In what anatomical triangle does the submandibular gland lie?
6. What nerves may be damaged during a submandibular gland excision?
7. Which vessels are usually encountered during the approach to the submandibular gland?
8. Which muscle separates the submandibular gland into deep and superficial lobes?
9. What are the attachments and nerve supply of this muscle?
10. Where do the submandibular ducts open inside the mouth?
11. What is the nerve supply to the submandibular gland?
12. Compare the acini type of the parotid, lingual and submandibular glands.
13. Salivary gland stones are most common in which gland?
14. Why is this?

Question 27

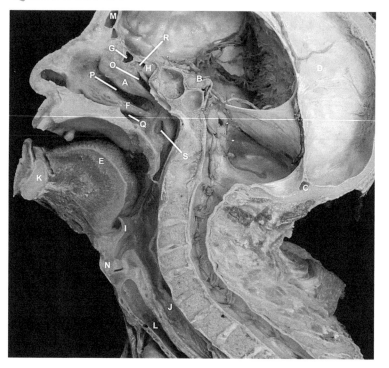

1. Name the structures labelled A–N.
2. At what age does structure M form?
3. Identify the structures labelled O–S.
4. With what do structures O–S communicate?
5. The pharynx can be divided into three parts. What are these parts called?
6. Describe the arrangement of the pharyngeal muscles.
7. What is the motor innervation of these muscles?
8. Describe the muscles of the palate.
9. What is the motor innervation of the palatal muscles?

Question 28

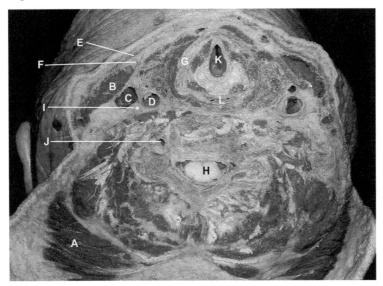

1. Identify the structures labelled A–L.
2. What vertebral level is this cross-section?
3. To which vertebral level does the isthmus of the thyroid gland correspond?
4. Describe the relationship of the thyroid gland to the layers of cervical fascia.
5. Describe the blood supply to the thyroid gland.
6. What structures are at risk of damage during ligation of these vessels during a thyroidectomy?
7. What are the consequences of this?
8. Describe the venous drainage of the thyroid gland.
9. Where are the parathyroid glands found?
10. What is the blood supply and venous drainage of the parathyroid glands?

Question 29

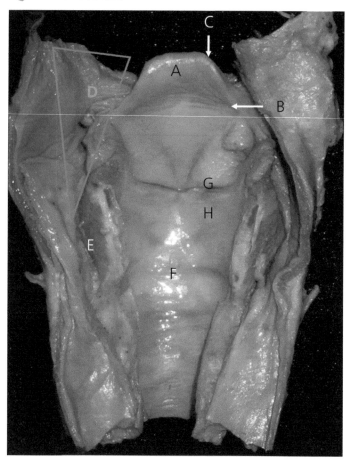

1. This is a larynx. Please orient the specimen.
2. What are the structures labelled A–C?
3. What is the name of the fossa marked with the blue triangle D?
4. What are the anatomical boundaries of this fossa?
5. Identify the muscle labelled E.
6. Why is muscle E so unique?
7. Describe the nerve supply of the muscles of the larynx.
8. What are the consequences of damage to these nerves?
9. Describe the likely position for a swallowed fishbone to lodge.
10. What membrane is marked by F?
11. What is the clinical relevance of point F?
12. What are the surface markings of this point?
13. What are the laryngoscopy appearances and the function of the two folds marked G and H?

Question 30

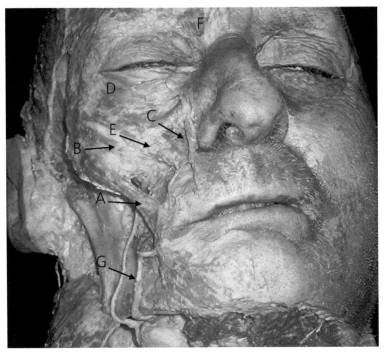

1. Name the muscles labelled A–F.
2. What is the structure labelled G?
3. What is the name of structure G as it ascends the face?
4. What is the nerve supply to the muscles of facial expression?
5. Does this nerve lie superficial or deep to these muscles?
6. Which muscles are supplied by the marginal mandibular branch of this nerve?
7. What is the clinical picture of an injury to this branch?
8. Which facial muscles cause the vertical and horizontal wrinkles in the glabella region?
9. Why is knowledge of this anatomy important to plastic surgeons?
10. Which cranial nerve provides sensation to the face?
11. What is a Bell's palsy?
12. What are the functional problems associated with this condition?

Question 19 – Answers

1. A – sternocleidomastoid
    B – trapezius
    C – omohyoid
    D – levator scapulae
    E – masseter
    F – splenius.
2. G – great auricular nerve
    H – accessory nerve.
3. I – external carotid artery
    J – facial artery
    K – superficial temporal artery
    L – maxillary artery.
4. The deep fascia of the neck is in several layers:
    The **investing layer of deep cervical fascia** is the most superficial layer and surrounds the entire neck. It is deep to the platysma muscle. It splits to enclose the sternocleidomastoid muscles anteriorly and the trapezius muscles posteriorly.
    The **prevertebral layer of deep cervical fascia** lies posteriorly and surrounds the vertebral column and the associated muscles (scalene muscles, longus colli, etc.).
    The **pretracheal layer of deep cervical fascia** lies anteriorly and surrounds the trachea, oesophagus and thyroid gland.
    The **carotid sheath** is another anterior (but paired) sheath of deep cervical fascia that lies on either side of the pretracheal fascia. It surrounds the carotid artery medially, the internal jugular vein laterally and the vagus nerve in between. It also contains the ansa cervicalis and some lymph nodes.
5. The posterior triangle of the neck is bordered:
    anteriorly by the posterior border of the sternocleidomastoid muscle
    posteriorly by the anterior border of the trapezius muscle
    inferiorly by the middle third of the clavicle.
    The roof is the investing layer of deep cervical fascia. The floor is the prevertebral fascia over the top of the following muscles:
    splenius capitis
    levator scapulae
    scalenus anterior

- scalenus medius
- scalenus posterior.

6. Sternocleidomastoid turns the head to the side opposite the muscle. To test the left sternocleidomastoid, ask the patient to turn their head to the right against resistance (hold your palm against their temple). Palpate for the contracting muscle. Trapezius elevates the scapula. To test the muscle, ask the patient to shrug their shoulders while you palpate the contracting muscle.

7. The contents of the posterior triangle of the neck are as follows:
   - **nerves:**
     - spinal accessory nerve
     - cervical plexus (lesser occipital, greater auricular, transverse cervical, supraclavicular)
     - brachial plexus (superior, middle and inferior trunks)
   - **arteries:**
     - third part of subclavian artery
     - transverse cervical artery (a branch of the thyrocervical trunk, a branch of the first part of the subclavian artery)
     - suprascapular artery (a branch of the thyrocervical trunk)
     - occipital artery – at the apex of the posterior triangle
   - **veins:**
     - external jugular vein.
   - **lymph nodes.**

8. Damage to the spinal accessory nerve in the posterior triangle results in paralysis of the ipsilateral trapezius.

9. The accessory nerve runs in a line from the transverse process of the atlas to the anterior border of trapezius, 5 cm above the clavicle.

10. The anterior triangle is bounded superiorly by the lower border of the mandible, posteriorly by the sternocleidomastoid and anteriorly by the midline.

11. The anterior triangle is subdivided into the submental, digastric (submandibular), carotid and muscular triangles.

12. The submental triangle is bounded by the anterior belly of digastric, the body of the hyoid and the midline. The digastric (or submandibular) triangle is bounded by the anterior and posterior bellies of digastric and the mandible. The carotid triangle is bounded by the sternocleidomastoid, the posterior belly of digastric and the omohyoid. The muscular triangle is bounded by the sternocleidomastoid, omohyoid and the midline.

Question 20 – Answers

1, 2. A – supraorbital foramen (or notch) – supraorbital nerve, artery and vein
   B – infraorbital foramen – infraorbital nerve, artery and vein
   C – mental foramen – mental nerve, artery and vein.
   Note how these three foramina lie roughly in a straight line that corresponds to the lateral limbus of the eye, a useful landmark for nerve blocks.

3. U – sphenoid
   V – mandible

W – zygoma
X – frontal bone
Y – nasal bone
Z – maxilla.

4. The superior orbital fissure is a slit-like foramen allowing communication between the middle cranial fossa and the orbit. From superior to inferior, the structures passing through this foramen are:
   lacrimal nerve
   frontal nerve
   (superior ophthalmic vein)
   trochlear nerve
   superior division of the oculomotor nerve
   nasociliary nerve
   inferior division of oculomotor nerve
   abducens nerve
   (inferior ophthalmic vein).

5–7. There are seven extraocular muscles: one eyelid elevator, four recti muscles and two oblique muscles. **Levator palpebrae superioris** originates from the sphenoid just above the tendinous ring and inserts into the tarsal plate of the upper eyelid. It elevates the upper eyelid. It has a dual nerve supply from the oculomotor nerve and sympathetic fibres that supply the autonomic component called Muller's muscle. **Superior rectus, inferior rectus, medial rectus** and **lateral rectus** originate from the tendinous ring (on the sphenoid) and attach into the sclera of the eye in positions corresponding to their names. Each muscle pulls the eye in the direction corresponding to its name, i.e. medial rectus pulls the eye medially, and lateral rectus pulls the eye laterally. Note that the superior and inferior recti do not pull the eye directly up or down, but rather they move slightly diagonally so that they slightly adduct the eye, i.e. superior rectus pulls the eye up and medially, and inferior rectus pulls the eye down and medially. This diagonal movement is corrected by the oblique muscles, which have a diagonal pull in the lateral direction (abduction). All of the recti are supplied by the oculomotor nerve, apart from the lateral rectus, which is supplied by the abducens nerve (remember 'abducens abducts the eye'). The **superior oblique** originates just above the tendinous ring and passes obliquely forwards and medially, passing through a pulley (trochlear) to then attach into the sclera posteriorly under the superior rectus. Its action is therefore to pull the eye inferiorly and laterally (down and out). The superior oblique is supplied by the trochlear nerve. The **inferior oblique** originates from the anterior medial orbital floor and inserts into the posterior lateral sclera. It pulls the eye superiorly and laterally (up and out). The inferior oblique is supplied by the oculomotor nerve.

8. The bony orbit is comprised of seven bones:
   frontal
   maxilla
   zygoma
   palatine

- lacrimal
- sphenoid
- ethmoid.

9. The oculomotor nerve supplies:
   - levator palpebrae superioris
   - medial rectus
   - superior rectus
   - inferior rectus
   - inferior oblique
   - parasympathetic fibres to the sphincter pupillae.

   An oculomotor nerve palsy therefore leaves the patient with a paralysed eye that looks **down and out** due to the unopposed pull of the lateral rectus (supplied by abducens nerve) and the superior oblique (supplied by the trochlear nerve). The pupil will be dilated due to the unopposed action of the sympathetic nerves on the dilator pupillae. The resulting strabismus will cause diplopia (double vision), which can cause discomfort, nausea and vomiting, but is rarely a significant problem with an oculomotor nerve palsy as the patient will have a simultaneous eyelid ptosis from paralysis of the levator palpebrae superioris. Note that the sympathetic fibres supplying Muller's muscle are inadequate to elevate the eyelid when acting alone.

Question 21 – Answers

1. A is the facial artery. This structure is easily identified by its tortuous course and can be palpated as it runs over the mandible, just anterior to the masseter. It often leaves a shallow groove in the bone that is easily palpated. Try feeling your own.
2. The facial artery originates from the external carotid artery.
3. B is the marginal mandibular nerve. Note how it runs over the palpable facial artery just as they cross the mandible. This is a useful place to identify the nerve surgically.
4. Damaging the marginal mandibular nerve (e.g. when exposing the facial vessels) will lead to paralysis of the ipsilateral depressor agularis oris muscle. The patient will not be able to depress the lower lip and will complain of an asymmetrical smile or biting their lower lip when eating.
5. C is the frontal (or temporal) branch of the facial nerve.
6. This lies in a relatively superficial position as it crosses the zygomatic arch and can be damaged here (e.g. during a face-lift).
7. As can be seen from the prosection, there are few interconnections between the frontal and zygomatic branches. For this reason, injury to the frontal branch at this level leads to a dense paralysis of the ipsilateral forehead. The patient is unable to elevate the affected eyebrow.
8,9. The facial nerve (or seventh cranial nerve) emerges from the junction of the pons and medulla. It traverses the posterior cranial fossa, runs within its own canal in the temporal bone, and then exits the skull at the stylomastoid foramen. Within the facial canal the facial nerve gives off the following:

greater petrosal nerve – these parasympathetic fibres then hitch a ride with the maxillary division of the trigeminal nerve (cranial nerve V2) to supply the lacrimal gland

- nerve to stapedius
- chorda tympani – these special sensory and parasympathetic fibres hitch a lift with the lingual nerve, a branch of the mandibular division of the trigeminal nerve (cranial nerve V3) to provide taste to the anterior two-thirds of the tongue and innervation to the submandibular and sublingual salivary glands
- auricular branch – supplies sensation to a small area of skin around the external auditory meatus.

After leaving the skull, the facial nerve gives off the posterior auricular nerve, which supplies the occipital belly of occipitofrontalis, gives off a branch that supplies the stylohyoid muscle and the posterior belly of digastric, and then enters the parotid gland. Within the gland the nerve divides into five branches – temporal, zygomatic, buccal, mandibular and cervical – which supply the muscles of facial expression. Most anatomy books describe five branches, but in fact the nerve has many branches that interconnect. For this reason, a cross-facial nerve graft does not leave a significant donor-side weakness, despite a major branch being cut. (The function of the facial nerve can be remembered by 'face, ear, taste, tear'.)

10. **temporal** – raise your eyebrows

   zygomatic – close your eyes tightly

   buccal – blow your cheeks out

   mandibular – show me your bottom teeth

   cervical – tense the skin on your neck and chin (platysma).

11. The parotid glands are paired salivary glands lying over the ramus and angle of the mandible. They are roughly triangular in shape. The edge of the parotid runs from the tragus of the ear in a line just below and parallel to the zygomatic arch to just overlap the posterior border of the masseter muscle. From here it arches back towards the angle of the mandible, around which it wraps. From this point it runs up, behind the ramus of the mandible and over the mastoid process, and curves forward around the inferior part of the auricle of the ear.

12. The parotid duct runs in the middle third of a line drawn from the intertragic notch (between tragus and anti-tragus of the ear) to the middle of the philtrum. It can be rolled over the tensed masseter.

13. The parotid duct empties saliva into the mouth at the papilla opposite the second maxillary molar tooth.

14. The buccal branch or branches of the facial nerve run alongside the parotid duct. In a patient with a cut or laceration to the cheek such as assault with a knife or glass, both structures can be damaged. As a general rule, a facial nerve laceration should be repaired if it is cut lateral to a line extending down from the lateral canthus of the eye. A cut medial to this line has similar outcomes with operative and conservative treatments. In patients with facial nerve injuries, laceration of the parotid duct should always be excluded by examining the papilla for signs of bleeding or bruising. The duct can be gently cannulated with a lacrimal probe and will be seen in the wound if a laceration exists.

Question 22 – Answers

1. A – helix
   B – anti-helix
   C – superior crus
   D – inferior crus
   E – triangular fossa
   F – scapha
   G – concha
   H – tragus
   I – intertragic notch
   J – anti-tragus
   K – lobule
   L – external acoustic meatus.

2. Six nerves contribute sensation to the ear:
   - **great auricular nerve** (branch of the cervical plexus) – supplies the inferior two-thirds of both sides of the ear
   - **lesser occipital nerve** (another branch of the cervical plexus) – supplies the superior one-third of the posterior ear
   - **auriculotemporal nerve** (branch of the mandibular division of trigeminal nerve) – supplies the superior third of the anterior ear (root and spine of helix)
   - **auricular branch of the vagus nerve** (Arnold's nerve) – supplies the concha and parts of the anti-helix anteriorly and posteriorly
   - **facial nerve** (the only somatic sensory branch) – via nerve branches from the tympanic plexus supplies part of the canal and tympanic membrane
   - **glossopharyngeal nerve** (Jacobson's nerve) – supplies a small portion of the external ear, being the main nerve to the middle ear.

3. The clinical consequences of this complex pattern of sensory supply are that pathology from a number of different sites can refer pain to the ear. The ear receives sensory fibres from four cranial nerves (trigeminal, facial, glossopharyngeal, vagus) and two spinal levels (C2, C3). Referred otalgia can be due to trigeminal neuralgia, or pathology of the molar teeth, parotid gland, temporomandibular joint, oropharynx, laryngopharynx, oesophagus or atlantoaxial joint. Any chronic ear pain with a normal ear examination must be assumed to be occult carcinoma of the head or neck unless proven otherwise (commonly base of tongue/tonsil).

4. The cervical plexus has four sensory branches (learned in this order they make a rhyme of sorts, which can help with memorising them):
   - lesser occipital
   - great auricular
   - transverse cervical
   - supraclavicular.

5. The ventral rami of C1–C4 form the cervical plexus, but only C2, C3 and C4 contribute to the sensory branches. The brachial plexus starts at C5 (and continues to T1). Therefore C1 has no sensory branch. The spinal level contributions are as follows:

lesser occipital C2
great auricular C2, C3
transverse cervical C2, C3
supraclavicular C3, C4.
6. Dermatomes:
C1 – there is no C1 dermatome
C2 – superoposterior scalp
C3 – upper neck and behind ear
C4 – lower neck down to clavicle.
7,8. The cervical plexus emerges through the prevertebral fascia at the posterior border of the sternocleidomastoid, approximately halfway along the muscle (more accurately at the level of the T6 transverse process). This is Erb's point.
9. This is a useful landmark to help find the accessory nerve during a neck dissection. The great auricular nerve is readily viewed when raising the subplatysma neck flaps. Erb's point is where the nerves disappear behind sternocleidomastoid. The accessory nerve is found 1 cm superior to this point and one plane deeper (i.e. deep to the investing layer of deep cervical fascia). The accessory nerve must be identified and preserved if possible when dissecting level 5 of a neck dissection. The cervical plexus sensory nerves are usually sacrificed.

Question 23 – Answers

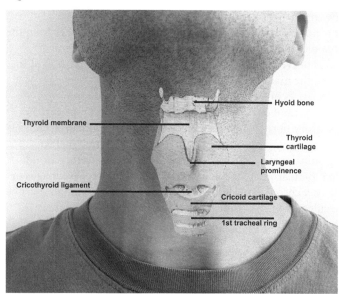

1. See figure.
2. During tracheostomy, the following layers are traversed:
skin
subcutaneous fat
platysma

- investing layer of deep cervical fascia
- strap muscles (sternohyoid and sternothyroid) – these are usually pulled aside rather than cut
- pretracheal fascia
- trachea.

3. The strap muscles (also known as the infrahyoid muscles) are a group of paired muscles that run in the anterior neck. They lie between the investing layer of deep cervical fascia and the pretracheal fascia. As their name describes, they are long, flat, strap-like muscles. The four muscles are called sternohyoid, thyrohyoid, sternothyroid and omohyoid.

4-6. Lying most superficially is **sternohyoid**. This attaches to the manubrium sternum inferiorly and the body of the hyoid bone superiorly. Its action is to depress the hyoid. The nerve supply is the ansa cervicalis. Lying deep to the sternohyoid in the superior neck is **thyrohyoid**. This attaches to the lower border of the body of the hyoid bone superiorly and the oblique line of the thyroid cartilage inferiorly. It depresses the hyoid and elevates the larynx. The muscle is supplied by C1 fibres from the cervical plexus that hitch-hike with the hypoglossal nerve. Lying deep to the sternohyoid in the lower neck is **sternothyroid**. This attaches inferiorly to the manubrium sternum and superiorly to the oblique line of the thyroid cartilage. It depresses the larynx. It is supplied by the ansa cervicalis. It can be seen, therefore, that sternothyroid and thyrohyoid together traverse the same path as sternohyoid, but they have an intermediate attachment on to the thyroid cartilage. Of course, they must lie deep to the sternohyoid as they have a deep attachment. Lying lateral to sternohyoid is **omohyoid**. This attaches inferiorly to the scapula and superiorly to the hyoid. It has an intermediate tendon that runs through a sling attached to the clavicle. The muscle therefore has a superior and an inferior belly separated by an intermediate tendon (similar to digastric). The action is to depress the hyoid. The nerve supply is the ansa cervicalis.

7. The strap muscles have a segmental blood supply (Mathes and Nahai type 4) via branches from the inferior and superior thyroid arteries.

8. Omohyoid is a useful landmark when performing a selective neck dissection as it marks the boundary between levels 3 and 4 in the anterior triangle. For example, if performing a neck dissection for a tongue squamous cell carcinoma (with no evidence of metastases), it is standard practice to dissect only levels 1, 2 and 3 of the neck as these are the most likely levels for tongue metastases. Levels 1–3 are also called a supraomohyoid neck dissection.

9.
- C1 = hard palate
- C2 = angle of mandible
- C3 = hyoid bone
- C4 = superior thyroid notch
- C5 = thyroid catilage
- C6 = cricoid cartilage
- C7 = upper tracheal rings.

Question 24 – Answers

1. 1 – superior thyroid artery
   2 – external carotid artery
   3 – lingual artery
   4 – facial artery
   5 – maxillary artery
   6 – middle meningeal artery
   7 – anterior cerebral artery
   8 – middle cerebral artery
   9 – superficial temporal artery
   10 – occipital artery
   11 – ascending pharyngeal artery
   12 – internal carotid artery
   13 – common carotid artery.
2. From inferior to superior the branches of the external carotid artery are:
   ascending pharyngeal
   superior thyroid
   lingual
   facial
   occipital
   posterior auricular
   superficial temporal
   maxillary.
3. The internal carotid artery has no branches in the neck, but after the cavernous sinus it divides into the anterior and middle cerebral and also gives off the smaller posterior communicating artery.
4. The common carotid artery bifurcates into the internal and external carotid arteries at the level of C4.
5. The maxillary artery is divided into three parts by its relation to the lateral pterygoid muscle. The first part (inferior to lateral pterygoid) has five branches:
   deep auricular artery
   anterior tympanic artery
   middle meningeal artery
   accessory meningeal artery
   inferior alveolar artery.
   The second part (behind lateral pterygoid) has four branches:
   deep temporal artery
   pterygoid artery
   masseteric artery
   buccal artery.
   The third part (superior to lateral pterygoid) has six branches:
   posterior superior alveolar artery
   infraorbital artery
   descending palatine artery
   artery of pterygoid canal

- pharyngeal artery
- sphenopalatine artery.

6. During surgery on the carotid artery (e.g. carotid endarterectomy) the following nerves are at risk of damage:
   - vagus nerve (including laryngeal nerve branches)
   - ansa cervicalis
   - hypoglossal nerve
   - sensory branches of the cervical plexus, especially the great auricular nerve
   - glossopharyngeal nerve
   - marginal mandibular branch of the facial nerve.

7. The vertebral artery is a branch of the first part of the subclavian artery.

8. The paired arteries pass between longus colli and scalenus anterior and ascend in the neck by passing through the foramina in the transverse processes (foramen transversarium) of the upper six cervical vertebrae, across the posterior arch of the atlas, and then enter the skull by passing through the foramen magnum.

9. The two vertebral arteries join to become the midline basilar artery as they reach the anterior surface of the medulla oblongata.

10. The basilar artery anastomoses with the internal carotid arteries to form the circle of Willis.

11. Subclavian **steal syndrome** is the occurrence of neurological impairment in the presence of a proximal subclavian artery stenosis. Subclavian **steal phenomenon** is found as an incidental finding in approximately 2% of the population but causes neurological symptoms in only approximately 5% of these patients. Subclavian steal occurs if there is a narrowing or occlusion (due to a number of different causes) of the subclavian artery proximal to the origin of the vertebral artery. There is reduced blood flow to the ipsilateral arm. To compensate, blood passes around the stenosis by going up the carotids, through the circle of Willis and then retrograde down the ipsilateral vertebral artery to supply the arm. Blood is therefore shunted or 'stolen' away from the brain to supply the arm. The left side is affected three times more commonly than the right side due to anatomical differences that make atherosclerosis more common. Neurological symptoms (e.g. vertigo, fainting, tinnitus, visual loss) occur when the ipsilateral limb is exercised. There is usually a marked difference in blood pressure between the two upper limbs.

Question 25 – Answers

1. The layers of the scalp are (from superficial to deep) (remember 'SCALP'):
   - skin
   - connective tissue
   - aponeurosis of occipitalis/frontalis muscles (also called galea)
   - loose connective (areolar) tissue
   - pericranium (periosteum of the skull).

2. The scalp receives blood from five paired arteries, two from the internal carotid and three from the external carotid. There is a ready anastomosis between the

systems. The **supraorbital** artery exits through the supraorbital foramen that lies in line with the lateral limbus of the iris. The **supratrochlear** artery exits the skull through the supratrochlear foramen or notch, which lies medial to the supraorbital foramen. Both of these anterior scalp vessels originate from the internal carotid artery system via the ophthalmic artery. The **occipital** artery lies posteriorly. The **superficial temporal** artery lies laterally in front of the ear. The **posterior auricular** artery lies laterally behind the ear. These posterior and lateral vessels originate from the external carotid artery.

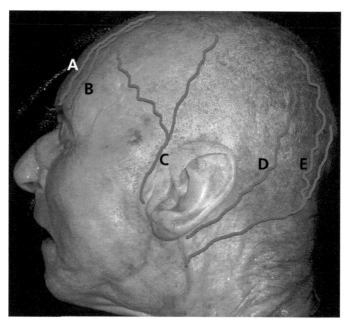

3. A – supratrochlear
    B – supraorbital
    C – superficial temporal dividing into anterior and posterior branches
    D – posterior auricular
    E – occipital.
4. The blood vessels and nerves run in the dense connective tissue below the skin (second layer). This layer also contains the hair follicles.
5. The scalp has a very rich blood supply to nourish the hair follicles and to regulate temperature, but the anatomy of the scalp also explains why lacerations here bleed so profusely. The blood vessels are embedded in the dense fibrous tissue beneath the skin. The vessel wall is attached firmly to this fibrous tissue, which reduces the normal vasospasm, retraction and contraction that are seen in cut vessels elsewhere. The bleeding vessels are held open.
6. Bleeding from scalp lacerations is best controlled by applying direct pressure to the wound and then by direct closure of the skin edge if possible. Ligation of individual vessels is rarely indicated.
7. Scalp flaps are usually raised in the subgaleal (subaponeurotic) plane. This loose areolar layer provides an easy plane for dissection with relatively few vessels or

fibrous attachments. Skin flaps raised more superficial to this plane are very bloody and adherent. Subpericranium flaps are sometimes used, but they have the disadvantage of leaving bare bone at the donor site. The pericranium is densely adherent to the underlying bone in the region of the sutures, making the dissection more difficult.

8. The venous drainage of the scalp closely follows the arteries of the same name (supratrochlear, supraorbital, superficial temporal, posterior auricular, occipital), but there are also valveless emissary veins that connect the superficial veins of the scalp with the diploic veins of the skull. These then drain into the intracranial venous sinuses.

9. This pattern of venous drainage has the rare potential to spread infections of the scalp into the diploic veins of the skull, causing osteomyelitis, or into the venous sinuses, causing thrombosis.

10. The nerve supply of the scalp is by branches of the cervical plexus, the trigeminal nerve and a posterior ramus nerve of C2 (remember 'Z-GLASS'):
    - zygomaticofrontal nerve (a branch of the maxillary division of the trigeminal nerve)
    - greater occipital nerve (a branch of the posterior ramus of C2)
    - lesser occipital nerve (cervical plexus C2)
    - auriculotemporal nerve (a branch of the mandibular division of the trigeminal nerve)
    - supraorbital nerve (a branch of the ophthalmic division of the trigeminal nerve)
    - supratrochlear nerve (another branch of the ophthalmic division of the trigeminal nerve).

Question 26 – Answers

1. This is a submandibular sialogram.
2. A – submandibular gland
    B – submandibular (Wharton's) duct.
3. The standard incision for submandibular gland surgery is 3 cm below the lower border of the mandible.
4. This is to avoid damaging the marginal mandibular branch of the facial nerve, which dips below the mandible on its path to supply the depressors of the lower lip.
5. The submandibular gland lies in the digastric or submandibular triangle.
6. The following nerves are at risk during submandibular gland surgery:
    - lingual nerve
    - nerve to mylohyoid
    - hypoglossal nerve
    - marginal mandibular nerve.
7. The facial artery and vein run over or through the gland and are usually ligated during submandibular gland surgery.
8. The mylohyoid muscle forms the floor of the mouth. The submandibular gland is wrapped around the free posterior border of this muscle, thus separating the gland into superficial and deep lobes.

9. This muscle attaches between the mylohyoid line on the internal border of the mandible and the hyoid. The nerve supply is a branch of the mandibular division of the trigeminal nerve (nerve to mylohyoid). Note that this nerve also supplies the anterior belly of digastric.
10. The submandibular (Wharton's) duct is 5 cm long and opens into the mouth beneath the tongue, on either side of the frenulum.
11. Secretion of saliva is stimulated by parasympathetic fibres that run in the chorda tympani branch of the facial nerve. The chorda tympani hitch-hikes with the lingual nerve (sensory branch of the mandibular division of trigeminal nerve). These fibres synapse in the submandibular ganglion, and then the postganglionic fibres pass directly into the gland.
12. The parotid gland is composed of predominantly serous acini, the submandibular gland has a mixture of serous and mucous acini, and the sublingual gland has almost all mucous acini.
13. Stones (sialolithiasis) are most commonly found in the submandibular gland and duct; 80% of stones occur here.
14. There are several theories as to why this is so:
   more viscous saliva (mucous acini)
   more alkaline saliva – leads to precipitation of calcium salts
   long, up-sloping Wharton's duct – gravity leads to accumulation of precipitate in the dependent part.

Question 27 – Answers

1. A – middle concha
   B – pituitary gland
   C – transverse sinus
   D – falx cerebri
   E – tongue
   F – inferior concha
   G – ethmoid sinus
   H – superior concha
   I – epiglottis
   J – oesophagus
   K – mandible
   L – trachea
   M – frontal sinus
   N – hyoid bone.
2. The frontal sinus is not present at birth but starts to appear as an air-filled space by about age 8 years. The sinus is not fully developed until puberty.
3. O – superior meatus
   P – middle meatus
   Q – inferior meatus
   R – sphenoethmoidal recess
   S – Eustachian (auditory) tube.
4. The superior meatus lies between the superior and middle conchae and communicates with the ethmoidal sinuses. The middle meatus lies between the

middle and inferior conchae and communicates with the frontal sinus through the frontonasal ducts and also the maxillary and ethmoidal sinuses. The inferior meatus lies below the inferior concha and communicates with the eye via the nasolacrimal duct. The sphenoethmoidal recess lies above the superior concha and communicates with the sphenoid sinus. The Eustachian tube links the middle ear to the nasopharynx.

5. The pharynx can be subdivided into the:
    - nasopharynx
    - oropharynx
    - laryngopharynx.

6. The muscles of the pharynx can be divided into three circular muscles:
    - superior constrictor
    - middle constrictor
    - inferior constrictor (whose upper fibres are called thyropharyngeus and the lower fibres are called cricopharyngeus)
    and three longitudinal muscles:
    - stylopharyngeus
    - salpingopharyngeus
    - palatopharyngeus.

    The constrictor muscles overlap each other posteriorly, with the lower muscle sitting outside the muscle above. This arrangement is analogous to three pint glasses stacked inside each other.

7. All of the muscles of the pharynx are supplied by the pharyngeal plexus (vagus and accessory nerves), apart from stylopharyngeus, which is supplied by the glossopharyngeal nerve.

8. There are five paired muscles that act on the soft palate:
    - tensor veli palatini
    - levator veli palatini
    - palatoglossus
    - palatopharyngeus
    - muscularis uvulae.

    The **tensor veli palatini** arises from the medial pterygoid plate, auditory tube and spine of sphenoid. It descends to the pterygoid hamulus and hooks around this bony point. From here the tendon opens into a broad aponeurosis, which blends with the aponeurosis of the opposite side. The hamulus changes the direction of pull of the muscle. Instead of elevating the soft palate it pulls it laterally, thus flattening and tensing the palate. The **levator veli palatini** arises from the petrous temple bone in front of the carotid canal. The paired muscles slope down in a V to attach to the soft palate. As the name implies, they elevate the palate, thus closing it against the posterior pharyngeal wall (Passavant's ridge). This prevents the passage of food into the nasopharynx during swallowing. Both the tensor and levator muscles also open the cartilaginous auditory tube to allow equalisation of middle ear pressure. The **palatoglossus** arises from the palate and inserts into the lateral portion of the tongue. These muscles form the anterior pillars of the fauces and form the junction between mouth and pharynx. Their action is to raise the tongue and depress the palate. The **palatopharyngeus** arises from both the hard and the soft palate. These two heads merge to form the posterior pillar of the fauces then insert into the pharynx and laryngeal cartilage. The action is to elevate the pharynx and larynx as well as depress the palate. The **muscularis uvulae** elevate the uvula.

9. All of the muscles of the palate are supplied by the pharyngeal plexus (vagus and accessory nerves), apart from the tensor veli palatini, which is supplied by the mandibular division of the trigeminal nerve (branch to medial pterygoid muscle).

Question 28 – Answers

1. A – trapezius
   B – sternocleidomastoid
   C – internal jugular vein
   D – carotid artery
   E – platysma
   F – investing layer of deep cervical fascia
   G – upper pole of thyroid gland
   H – spinal cord
   I – vagus nerve
   J – vertebral artery
   K – larynx
   L – pharynx (compressed).

2. This cross-section is at the C4/C5 level. (The carotid artery has not bifurcated yet (C4) and the vocal cords are just visible in the arytenoid cartilage.)

3. The isthmus of the thyroid gland is at the level of the C7 vertebra.

4. The thyroid gland lies within its own covering of connective tissue – the thyroid fascia. This is within the pretracheal fascia, which surrounds the larynx and pharynx as well. The pretracheal and prevertebral fascia lie within the investing layer of deep cervical fascia.

5. The thyroid gland is supplied bilaterally by the superior and inferior thyroid arteries. The superior thyroid artery is a branch of the external carotid artery and supplies the upper pole. The inferior thyroid artery is a branch of the thyrocervical trunk and supplies the lower pole. About 3% of the population have a thyroidea ima artery, a midline artery from the brachiocephalic trunk that supplies the isthmus of the gland.

6,7. The recurrent laryngeal nerve runs close (usually posterior) to the inferior thyroid artery and is at risk of damage during ligation of this vessel. This nerve supplies all the muscles of the larynx, except for the cricothyroid muscle. Damage to this nerve leads to paralysis of the ipsilateral vocal cord. Bilateral partial recurrent laryngeal nerve palsy can lead to fatal occlusion of the airway (see the question on the larynx, p. 69). The external laryngeal nerve runs close to the superior thyroid artery and is at risk of damage during ligation of this vessel. This nerve supplies the cricothyroid muscle, and damage to it will manifest itself as a loss of timbre of the voice (monotone speech).

8. The thyroid gland is usually drained bilaterally by three veins:
   - superior thyroid vein

middle thyroid vein

inferior thyroid vein.

The superior and middle veins empty into the internal jugular vein on that side. The inferior vein empties into the brachiocephalic vein.

9. There are two parathyroid glands on each side of the neck. They usually lie deep to the lateral aspect of the thyroid gland. The superior glands have a more constant position, level with the first tracheal ring. The inferior glands are more variably located, not always behind the inferior pole of the thyroid gland; they are sometimes found within the thyroid gland itself or rarely in the mediastinum.

10. All of the parathyroid glands are supplied by the inferior thyroid arteries, with the superior glands also receiving blood from the superior thyroid arteries. Venous drainage is via the superior, middle and inferior thyroid veins.

Question 29 – Answers

1. The epiglottis is superior, arising from the anterior surface. The tracheal rings are inferior. The specimen shown is therefore viewed from the incised posterior side, i.e. we are looking at the front of the larynx from the inside.

2. A – epiglottis

    B – aryepiglottic fold

    C – vallecula.

3. D is piriform fossa.

4. This is bounded medially by the aryepiglottic fold and laterally by the thyroid cartilage and the thyrohyoid membrane.

5. E is the posterior cricoarytenoid muscle.

6. The posterior cricoarytenoid is the most important muscle in the body as it is the only abductor of the vocal cords.

7. All the intrinsic muscles of the larynx are supplied by the recurrent laryngeal nerve, except the cricothyroid muscle, which is supplied by the external laryngeal nerve.

8. A complete recurrent laryngeal nerve palsy leaves the paralysed cords in mid-adduction, i.e. between full abduction and adduction. Partial recurrent laryngeal nerve injuries weaken the abductors more than the adductors, thus leaving the cords in the closed (adducted) position. This phenomenon is poorly understood, but in the case of bilateral partial recurrent laryngeal nerve palsy life-threatening airway obstruction can occur and may necessitate a tracheostomy. Clinically a recurrent laryngeal nerve palsy leaves the patient with a hoarse voice, but in the unilateral scenario the patient is still able to phonate by adducting the functioning cord against the paralysed cord. External laryngeal nerve palsy leaves the patient unable to tense their vocal cord and therefore unable to change the pitch of their voice (sometimes referred to as 'singer's nerve').

9. Food usually passes laterally through the piriform fossae rather than over the epiglottis. For this reason a fishbone is most likely to catch in the valleculae or piriform fossae.

10. F is the cricothyroid membrane.
11. This is the site for performing a cricothyroidotomy (not a tracheostomy, which is inserted through the tracheal rings).
12. Clinically this is the gap palpated just inferior to the laryngeal prominence (Adam's apple).
13. **G is the vestibular fold**, or false cords. These have a minimal role in phonation but are important in protecting the airway. The patient with a resected epiglottis has the same risk of aspiration as patients with an epiglottis due to these folds. They are thought to produce the purring noise in cats. These are fixed structures and composed of mucosa overlying the vestibular ligament. They are pink in life due to blood flow in the mucosa. **H is the vocal fold** (vocal cord), or true cords. They are responsible for sound production. They are mobile structures and composed of mucosa over the vocal ligament. They are white in appearance because they are relatively avascular.

Question 30 – Answers

1. A – zygomaticus major
   B – zygomaticus minor
   C – levator labii superioris alaeque nasi
   D – orbicularis oculi
   E – levator labii superioris
   F – procerus.
2. G is the facial artery.
3. The facial artery changes its name to the angular artery as it ascends towards the medial canthus of the eye.
4. The muscles of the face are supplied by the facial nerve.
5. Most of the facial muscles lie superficial to the facial nerve (i.e. they are supplied on their deep surface). Three muscles lie deep to the nerve. They are buccinator, mentalis and levator anguli oris.
6. The marginal mandibular branch of the facial nerve supplies the mentalis, depressor anguli oris and depressor labii inferioris.
7. Injury to this nerve leads to an inability to depress the lower lip and angle of the mouth. This causes an obvious alteration to the appearance of the smile and can also lead to frequent biting of the lower lip.
8. Skin wrinkles are caused by the contraction of underlying muscles that are oriented in a direction perpendicular to the wrinkle. In the glabella region the vertical wrinkles are caused by the action of corrugator supercilii and the horizontal wrinkles are due to procerus.
9. These frown lines are frequently the target of botulinum toxin injection for aesthetic improvement of the forehead. Knowledge of the underlying muscle anatomy is important to accurately administer the botulinum toxin to provide reliable results and to avoid unwanted paralysis of nearby muscles (e.g. levator palpebrae superioris, which would cause eyelid ptosis).
10. The trigeminal (fifth) nerve provides sensation to the face.

11. A Bell's palsy is a mononeuropathy affecting the facial nerve. This is a diagnosis of exclusion and should be made only after other causes have been ruled out (e.g. trauma, infection, stroke, tumour). The result is a varying degree of paralysis of the facial muscles.
12. Aesthetic and functional deficits can result:
    - loss of facial animation, e.g. smiling – this is not only an aesthetic deficit, as one of the main functions of the face is non-verbal communication
    - loss of blink/eye closure due to paralysis of orbicularis oculi – dry eyes, exposure keratitis and corneal ulceration may result; eyelid opening is maintained as the levator is supplied by the oculomotor nerve
    - closure of ipsilateral nasal airway due to paralysis of the nasal dilator muscles.
    - drooling of saliva and loss of oral competence due to paralysis of orbicularis oris and mouth sphincter function
    - food bolus pooling in cheeks– the buccinators help push food out of the cheek pouches and into the path of the teeth during chewing
    - unilateral hyperacusis due to paralysis of stapedius.

3

Question 31

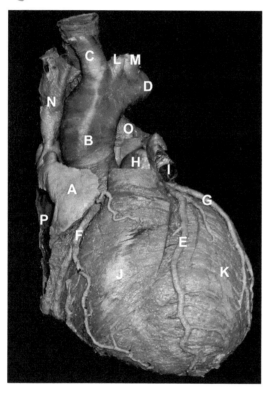

1. Name the structures labelled A–P.
2. Demonstrate the surface markings of the heart.
3. What are the surface markings of the tracheal carina?
4. What are the landmarks for inserting a chest drain?
5. What layers would you go through when inserting a chest drain?
6. In which of these planes do the intercostal vessels run?
7. Compare the muscle layers of the chest wall with those of the abdominal wall.
8. In which direction are the external intercostal muscle fibres oriented?
9. What are the surface markings of the parietal pleura?
10. Are there any areas where the pleural cavity is not protected by the rib cage?

Question 32

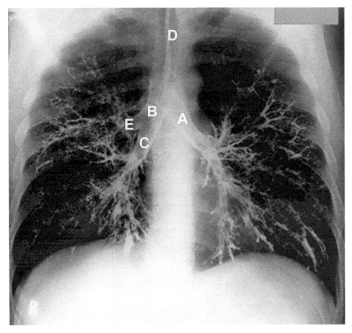

1. What investigation is this?
2. What are the structures labelled A–E?
3. Which of the main bronchi (right or left) would an inhaled foreign object choose in preference, and why?
4. How many lobes do the lungs have?
5. How many bronchopulmonary segments does each lung have?

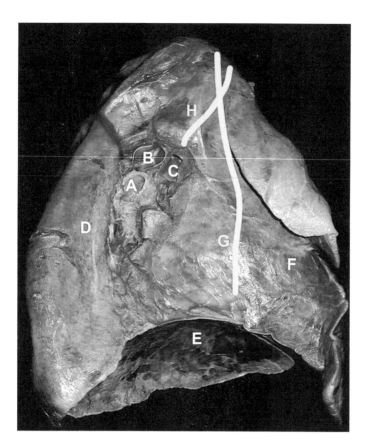

6. From which side is this lung?
7. What structures cause impressions D–F on the lung?
8. What nerves run in the positions marked G and H?
9. What are the structures labelled A–C?
10. What are the surface markings of the lung fissures?

Question 33

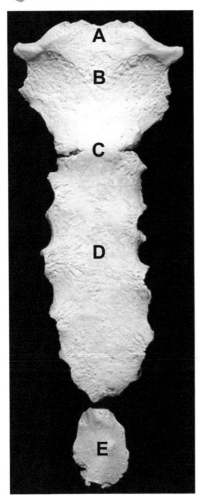

1. What is this bone?
2. What are the parts of this bone labelled A–E?
3. To which thoracic vertebrae levels do the different parts of this bone correspond?
4. What is the motor nerve supply to the diaphragm?
5. From what spinal levels does this nerve arise?
6. What nerves supply sensation to the diaphragm?
7. From what spinal levels do these nerve arise?
8. What is the clinical relevance of this sensory supply to the diaphragm?
9. What is the blood supply to the diaphragm?
10. What structures pass through the diaphragm, and at which levels?
11. What are the surface markings of these openings?

Question 34

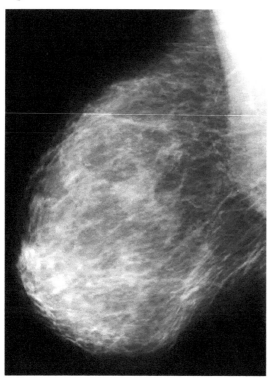

1. What is this investigation?
2. Describe the anatomy of the breast parenchyma.
3. Describe the pattern of lymphatic drainage of the breast.
4. What are the boundaries of the breast?
5. What is the blood supply to the breast?
6. What is the sensory nerve supply to the breast?
7. What nerve supplies sensation to the nipple?
8. The breast is a modified type of which kind of common skin gland?

Question 35

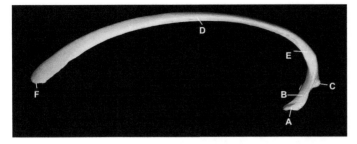

1. What bone is this?
2. What are the names of the points labelled A–E?
3. What attaches to the point labelled F?
4. What articulates with point C?
5. What movements do the ribs make during respiration?

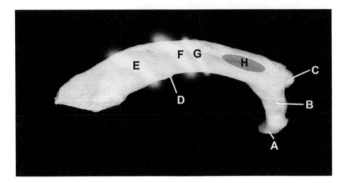

6. What bone is this?
7. Identify the bony points labelled A–D.
8. What attaches to the point labelled D?
9. What structures cause the grooves E and F?
10. What structure runs in position G?
11. What structures run above and below point B?
12. What bone articulates with point A?
13. What muscle attaches at point H?

Question 36

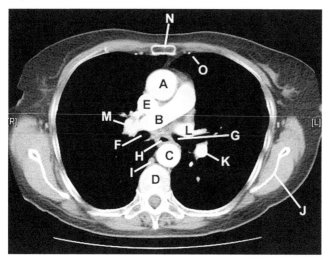

1. At what vertebral level is this computed tomography (CT) scan?
2. Identify the structures labelled A–O on this CT scan.
3. What is the blood supply to the oesophagus?
4. What constrictions occur in the oesophagus (as seen during oesophagoscopy)?
5. Through what structures would a needle pass during subclavian vein cannulation?
6. What structures are at risk during subclavian vein cannulation?

Question 37

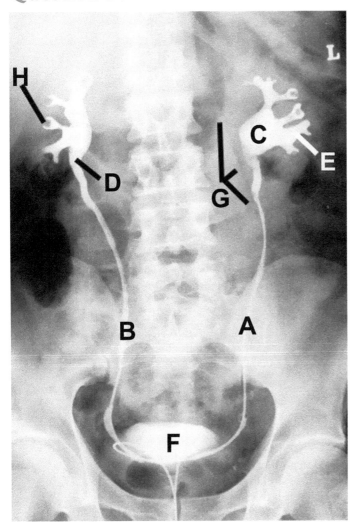

1. What is this investigation?
2. Identify the structures labelled A–F.
3. What structure forms the faint line marked by G?
4. What causes the cup-shaped impression labelled H?
5. Describe the course of the ureters. What are their relations?
6. What is the blood supply of the ureters?
7. What causes constrictions of the ureter as seen on intravenous urography?
8. What is the composition of different types of renal calculus?
9. What is the most common type of urinary tract calculus?

Question 38

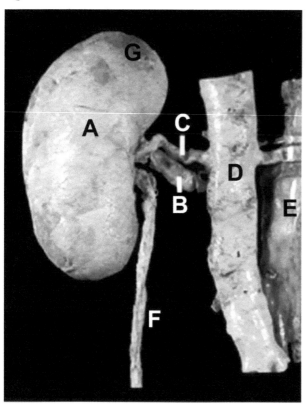

1. What is the name of this organ labelled A?
2. Identify the structures labelled B–F.
3. What organ is related to position G?
4. What is the usual order of structures at the hilum of this organ?
5. Therefore, from which side is this organ?
6. At what vertebral levels does this organ lie, and what are its fascial layers?
7. What are the posterior relations of this organ?
8. Is this organ intraperitoneal or retroperitoneal?
9. What is the lymphatic drainage of this organ?
10. Describe the internal structure of this organ
11. What is the functional unit of this organ?
12. How many of these units are present?

Question 39

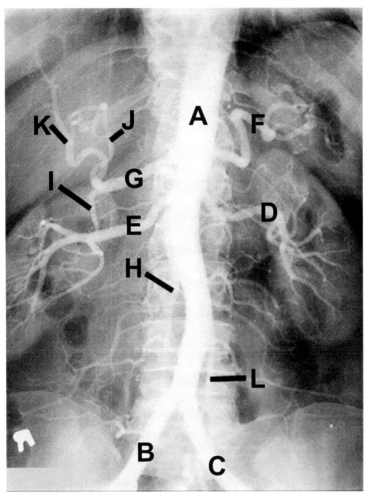

1. What is this investigation?
2. Identify the vessels labelled A–L.
3. Describe the course of the abdominal aorta.
4. Name the branches and describe the level at which they arise.
5. What is the definition of an aneurysm?
6. What is the difference between a false and a true aneurysm?
7. Describe the course of the inferior vena cava in the abdomen, including its relations to the aorta.
8. Describe the tributaries, relations and course of the portal vein.

Question 40

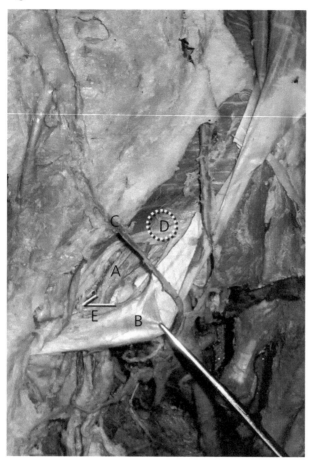

1. This is a dissected specimen of the inguinal region. Identify the structures labelled A–C.
2. What is represented by the circle D and the V-shaped E?
3. From which side of the body is the specimen?
4. What is the inguinal canal?
5. What are the boundaries of the inguinal canal?
6. What runs through the inguinal canal?
7. What is the mid-inguinal point, and what is found here?
8. What is the midpoint of the inguinal ligament, and what is found here?
9. What are the layers of the spermatic cord and scrotum, and from which layers of the abdominal wall are they derived?
10. What are the contents of the spermatic cord?
11. What is the fate of the right and left testicular veins?
12. What is the clinical relevance of this?

Question 41

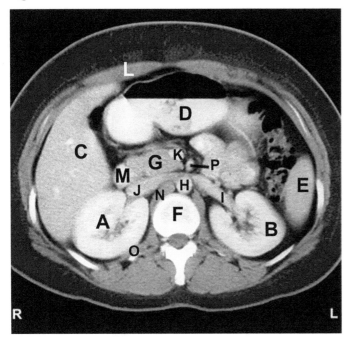

1. What is this investigation, and through which vertebral level is it taken?
2. Name the structures labelled A–P.
3. What is the transpyloric plane, and what structures lie at this level?
4. Describe the blood supply to the stomach.
5. Describe the venous drainage of the stomach.
6. Where are the sites of portosystemic anastomoses?
7. Describe the origin, path and branches of the superior mesenteric artery.
8. Describe the blood supply of the duodenum.
9. Describe the blood supply of the pancreas.
10. What is the lumbar plexus, and to what muscle is it related?
11. What nerves arise from the lumbar plexus?

Question 42

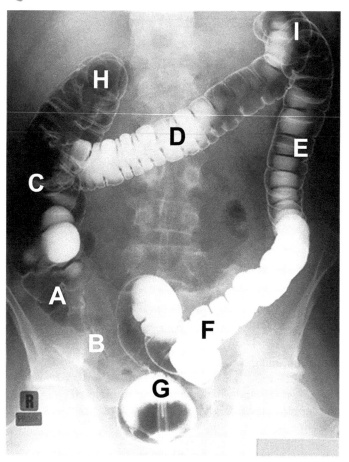

1. What is this investigation? Name the labelled parts.
2. Which parts of the colon are retroperitoneal?
3. Describe the blood supply of the colon.
4. Describe the peritoneal relations of the rectum.
5. Which abdominal and pelvic structures are intraperitoneal, and which are retroperitoneal?
6. What characteristics will help distinguish between jejunum and ileum?
7. What characteristics will help distinguish between large bowel and small bowel?

Question 43

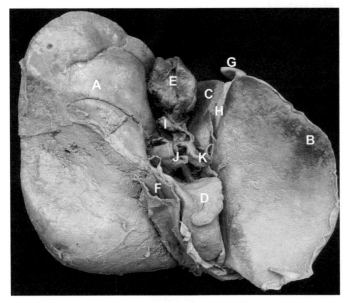

1. What organ is this, and from which angle is the photograph taken?
2. Name the different lobes labelled A–D.
3. What are the structures labelled E–K?
4. What is Calot's triangle? What forms the boundaries, and what are the contents?
5. What is the epiploic foramen (of Winslow)?
6. What are the boundaries of the epiploic foramen?
7. A finger can be inserted into the epiploic foramen and squeezed against a thumb anteriorly. What is the name of this procedure?
8. What structures are squeezed?
9. What is this used for?

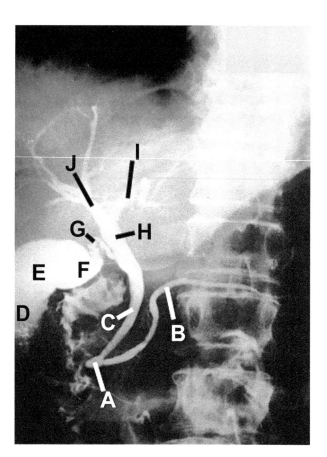

10. What is this investigation?
11. Name the parts labelled A–J.
12. Where does the common bile duct enter the bowel?
13. What anatomical structure controls the secretion of bile?

Question 44

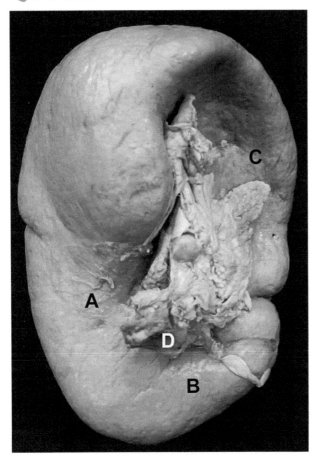

1. What is this organ?
2. From which side of the body is this?
3. What adjacent organs have left the impressions shown by A–D?
4. Is this organ normally palpable? If not, how much bigger must it be before it is palpable?
5. In the supine person, what part of the abdomen is the most dependent?
6. What clinical significance does this have?
7. What structures make up the rectus sheath? Is this the same for the entire length?
8. Through which layers would a surgeon cut during a midline laparotomy incision?

Question 45

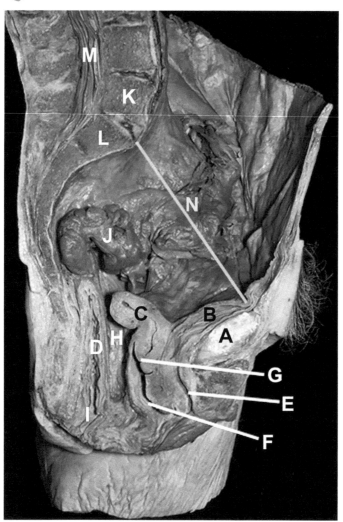

1. Is this a male or female pelvis?
2. Name the structures labelled A–M.
3. What is the name of the aperture N?
4. Describe the different parts of the urethra in the male.
5. Which part of the urethra is responsible for control of the flow of urine?
6. Which is the most dilatable part of the urethra?
7. Which is the least dilatable part of the urethra?

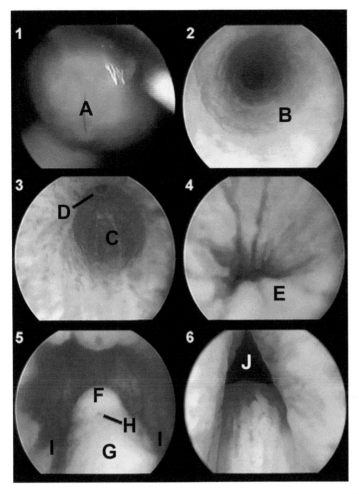

8. This is a series of photographs taken during a cystoscopy. Is this from a male or female?
9. Identify the structures labelled A–J.
10. What structure(s) open into point H, and what is their function?
11. What structure(s) open into point I?

Question 46

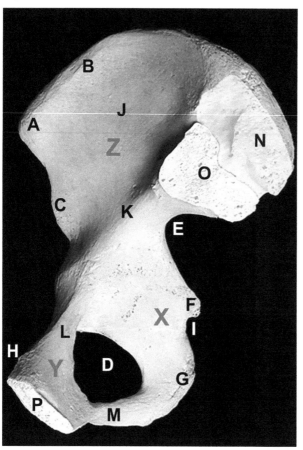

1. What bone is this?
2. Identify the points labelled A–M.
3. What are the names of the three parts labelled X, Y and Z that form this bone?
4. Where do these three bones meet?
5. What attaches between points A and H?
6. What is represented by the blue shading at points O and P?
7. What muscle originates from point J?

3 THORAX AND ABDOMEN – ANSWERS

Question 31 – Answers

1. A – right auricle
   B – ascending aorta
   C – brachiocephalic trunk
   D – arch of aorta
   E – left anterior descending coronary artery (anterior interventricular artery)
   F – right coronary artery
   G – marginal artery
   H – pulmonary trunk
   I – left pulmonary artery
   J – right ventricle
   K – left ventricle
   L – left carotid artery
   M – left subclavian artery
   O – left main bronchus
   P – inferior vena cava.

2.

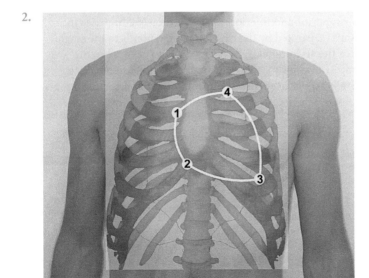

1 – lower border of the third costal cartilage at the right edge of the sternum

2 – lower border of the sixth costal cartilage at the right of the sternum

3 – fifth intercostal space in the mid-clavicular line

4 – second intercostal space, 2 cm to the left of the sternum.

Draw a slightly curved line between these four points.

3. The trachea bifurcates into left and right main bronchi just below the level of the manubriosternal junction.

4. A chest drain is usually inserted in the fourth intercostal space in the anterior axillary line, just superior to the fifth rib (this avoids damaging the intercostal vessels that run in the upper part of the intercostal space, just inferior to the corresponding rib).

5. The drain passes through:
   skin
   subcutaneous fat
   deep fascia
   serratus anterior muscle
   external intercostal muscle
   internal intercostal muscle
   innermost intercostal muscle
   endothoracic fascia
   parietal pleura.

6. The intercostal neurovascular bundle runs in the plane between the internal intercostal and the innermost intercostal muscles in the order vein–artery–nerve from superior to inferior.

7. The muscles of the chest wall can be divided into three layers, just as the abdominal wall musculature can be. The outer layer comprises the external intercostals (separated by the ribs) and corresponds to the single external oblique of the abdomen. The outer layer of the chest wall also includes the serratus posterior superior and inferior. The middle layer comprises the internal intercostals (separated by the ribs) and corresponds to the single internal oblique of the abdominal wall. The inner layer comprises the transversus thoracis (anteriorly), subcostals (posteriorly) and innermost intercostals (laterally). This layer corresponds to the transversus abdominis layer of the abdomen. The neurovascular plane of both regions is between the middle and inside layers.

8. The external intercostal muscle fibres are oriented in the same direction as the external oblique fibres, i.e. running down and forward.

9. The parietal pleura provide the lining of the thoracic cavity. The pleural cavity extends 3 cm above the first rib anteriorly (but level with the raised posterior aspect of the first rib). The edge of the pleura extends down from the sternoclavicular joint to meet the pleura of the other side at the second rib. At the fourth rib level the left side moves lateral to the sternum, whereas the right side continues down the midline. At the sixth rib both sides turn laterally. At the eighth rib they reach the mid-clavicular line and the mid-axillary line over the tenth rib. The lower border varies according to the position of the diaphragm but lies above the lower border of the rib cage. The pleural line crosses the

twelfth rib just lateral to the erector spinae and then passes horizontally to the T12 vertebra.

10. The pleural cavity extends above the upper border of the first rib anteriorly. Posteriorly the pleural cavity extends below the lower border of the twelfth rib for a short distance on either side of the midline.

Question 32 – Answers

1. This is a contrast bronchogram.
2. A – left main bronchus
   B – right main bronchus
   C – intermediate bronchus
   D – trachea
   E – right upper lobe bronchus.
3. The right main bronchus is larger in diameter and forms less of an angle with the trachea than the left. For this reason a foreign body will tend to fall down the right side.
4. The right lung has three lobes – upper, middle and lower. The left lung has two lobes – upper and lower.
5. The right lung has ten segments (three in the upper lobe, two in the middle lobe, five in the lower lobe). The left lung has nine or ten segments (four or five in the upper lobe, five in the lower lobe).
6. This is the medial aspect of the left lung. (The flat diaphragmatic base faces down, while the thinner, sharper anterior border faces forwards.)
7. D – aorta
   E – diaphragm
   F – heart.
8. G – phrenic nerve (anteriorly)
   H – vagus nerve (posteriorly).
9. A – left main bronchus
   B – pulmonary artery
   C – pulmonary vein.
10. Both lungs have an oblique fissure that extends from the spinous process of the T2 vertebra posteriorly to the sixth costal cartilage anteriorly. The right lung also has a horizontal fissure that lies under the fourth rib.

Question 33 – Answers

1. This is the sternum.
2. A – jugular notch
   B – manubrium
   C – sternal angle (of Louis)
   D – body
   E – xiphoid process.

3.   sternal notch – disc between T2 and T3
    manubrium – T3 to T4
    sternal angle (of Louis) – disc between T4 and T5
    body of sternum – T5 to T8
    xiphisternum – T9.

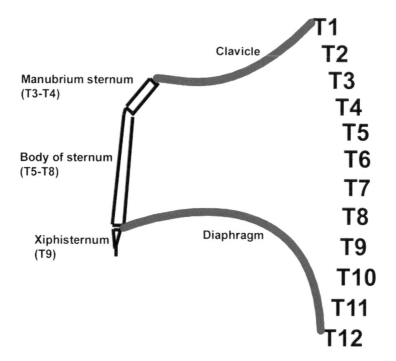

4. The right and left phrenic nerves are the motor supply to the diaphragm.

5. The phrenic nerves arise from the C3–C5 spinal levels ('C3–C5 keep the diaphragm alive').

6,7. The phrenic nerve (C3–C5) provides sensation to the central part of the diaphragm, while the intercostal nerves T5–T11 and subcostal T12 provide sensation to the peripheral part.

8. Irritation of the central part of the diaphragm (e.g. from a bleeding splenic laceration) is felt as referred pain in the dermatome of the phrenic nerve roots – C3–C5 – i.e. the shoulder. Irritation to the peripheral parts of the diaphragm is felt more locally.

9. The diaphragm is supplied by the following arteries:
  superior and inferior phrenic arteries from the aorta
  musculophrenic branches of the internal mammary artery
  small contribution from the intercostal arteries to the peripheral parts of the diaphragm.

10. There are three large openings in the diaphragm. At the level of T8 is the caval opening, which allows passage of the inferior vena cava, the right phrenic nerve and lymphatic vessels. At the level of T10 is the oesophageal hiatus,

which allows passage of the oesophagus, vagus nerve, left gastric vessels and lymphatics. At the level of T12 is the aortic hiatus, which allows passage of the aorta, azygous vein and thoracic duct. This is actually an aperture posterior to the diaphragm rather than a true hole within it.

11. T8 – xiphisternal junction

   T10 – seventh costal cartilage

   T12 – just above transpyloric plane.

Question 34 – Answers

1. This is a mammogram.
2. The female breast is composed of an arrangement of gland and duct tissue, with a variable amount of intervening fat. The terminal duct lobular units produce milk. These drain into approximately 10–20 lactiferous ducts that converge on the nipple in a radial distribution. Each duct has a separate opening in the nipple. The glandular breast is supported by fibrous septae known as the suspensory ligaments of Astley Cooper, which are condensations of fascia that run between the dermis of the breast skin and the posterior capsule of the breast. These ligaments maintain the shape of the young breast but become attenuated with age, leading to ptosis.
3. As a general rule, the lateral part of the breast drains to the axillary lymph nodes, while the medial breast drains to the internal thoracic nodes. There are multiple valveless channels connecting these systems, however, which allow lymph to flow in both directions depending on external pressure and gravity. Most lymph seems to drain into the ipsilateral axillary basin via the anterior axillary nodes and central axillary nodes, through to the apical axillary nodes. Some lymph drains to infraclavicular and supraclavicular nodes, subscapular, interpectoral, rectus sheath, contralateral breast and even mediastinal nodes. Intramammary lymph nodes are frequently found, especially in the upper outer quadrant of the breast.
4. The base of the breast is circular and extends from the lateral border of the sternum to the mid-axillary line, from the second rib down to the sixth rib.
5. The breast receives blood from four sources:
   medially from branches of the internal mammary artery
   laterally from branches of the lateral thoracic artery
   deeply through perforators from the pectoralis major muscle (thoracoacromial trunk)
   inferiorly/laterally from branches of the intercostal arteries.
6. The breast skin is supplied by:
   supraclavicular branches of the cervical plexus (C3 and C4)
   lateral cutaneous branches of the anterior thoracic intercostal nerves
   anterior perforating cutaneous branches of the intercostal nerves
   intercostobrachial nerve.
7. The nipple is supplied by the fourth intercostal nerve.
8. The breast is a modified apocrine sweat gland.

Question 35 – Answers

1. This is the superior aspect of a typical rib from the right side (this happens to be the eighth rib). Note the upper surface is blunt, whereas the inferior border has a sharp edge, lateral to the costal groove. The neurovascular bundle runs behind this sharp edge.
2. A – head
   B – neck
   C – tubercle
   D – shaft
   E – angle.
3. The costal cartilage.
4. This is the tubercle of the rib and has a facet for articulation with the transverse process of the corresponding vertebra (e.g. if this is the fourth rib, then the tubercle would articulate with the transverse process of the T4 vertebra).
5. During inspiration, contraction of the intercostal muscles causes the middle of the ribs to rise upwards (bucket-handle movement). This increases the transverse diameter of the chest. Movement of the ribs at the costovertebral joints also allows the anterior ends of the ribs to rise upwards (pump-handle movement), thus increasing the anteroposterior diameter of the chest.
6. This is a right first rib. (Note how flat, small and tightly curved it is. The superior surface has the grooves.)
7. A – head
   B – neck
   C – tubercle
   D – scalene tubercle.
8. The scalene tubercle provides attachment for the scalenus anterior muscle.
9. E – subclavian vein
   F – subclavian artery.
10. The T1 nerve root runs in direct contact with the shaft of the rib, with the fibres of the C8 nerve root running above it. These nerve roots merge to form the inferior trunk of the brachial plexus.
11. The C8 nerve root runs above the neck of the first rib and the T1 nerve root runs below the neck. Both structures then pass above the shaft of the first rib (position G).
12. This is the head of the first rib and has a facet for articulation with the T1 vertebra.
13. The scalenus medius muscle attaches to the first rib here.

Question 36 – Answers

1. This CT scan is at the level of the pulmonary arteries. It is therefore at the T5 vertebral level.
2. A – ascending aorta
   B – right pulmonary artery
   C – descending aorta
   D – body of T5 vertebra
   E – superior vena cava

F – right main bronchus

G – left main bronchus

H – oesophagus

I – azygous vein

J – left scapula

K – left lower lobe pulmonary artery

L – left pulmonary vein

M – right pulmonary vein

N – sternum

O – left internal mammary artery.

3.   superior part – inferior thyroid arteries

    middle part – oesophageal branches of descending aorta

    lower part – left gastric artery and inferior phrenic artery.

4. The following structures cause a constriction in the oesophagus (from superior to inferior):

    upper oesophageal sphincter

    arch of aorta presses against left lateral surface of oesophagus

    left main bronchus

    diaphragmatic hiatus.

5. During subclavian vein cannulation the needle passes through:

    skin

    subcutaneous fat

    deep fascia

    clavicular head of pectoralis major

    clavipectoral fascia

    subclavius

    subclavian vein wall.

6. At risk of damage are:

    subclavian artery

    phrenic nerve

    apex of lung

    thoracic duct (on left side).

Question 37 – Answers

1. This is a retrograde pyelogram. (Note the contrast catheters inserted through the urethra and bladder and into the ureters. This is not an intravenous urogram (IVU), in which the contrast is given via a vein and then filtered by the kidneys. The appearance of the kidneys and ureters is similar in both investigations.)

2. A – left ureter

B – right ureter

C – left renal pelvis

D – right pelvi-ureteric junction

E – calyx

F – bladder.

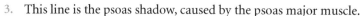

3. This line is the psoas shadow, caused by the psoas major muscle.

4. The renal papillae project into the minor calyces, causing this characteristic shape. The minor calyces unite to form two or three major calyces, which then empty into the renal pelvis.

5. The ureters start at the renal pelvis – the most posterior of the renal hilum structures (vein, artery, pelvis from anterior to posterior). They are retroperitoneal for their entire course, and there is an equal length of ureter in the abdomen and in the pelvis. The abdominal ureter descends almost vertically downwards, anterior to the psoas major muscle, just overlapping the transverse processes of the lumbar vertebrae. Each ureter is crossed anteriorly by the gonadal artery and vein. The genitofemoral nerve passes behind the ureter (which explains the referred pain to the testes with ureteric calculi). At the pelvic brim, the ureters pass anterior to the external iliac artery (ureter, artery, vein from anterior to posterior). The left ureter has the apex of the sigmoid mesocolon as its anterior relation at the pelvic brim. The pelvic ureter then descends posteroinferiorly on the lateral pelvic wall, anterior to the branches of the internal iliac arteries, and then curves anteromedially to enter the posterolateral surface of the bladder. Just before entering the bladder the ureter is crossed anteriorly by the vas deferens in the male or the uterine artery in the female.

6. **superior** – ureteric branches of the renal arteries

   middle – branches of the gonadal arteries

   inferior – branches of the common and external iliac arteries

   pelvic – branches of the internal iliac and vesical arteries.

7. pelvic-ureteric junction

   ureter changes direction as it crosses the pelvic brim

   crossing of the gonadal artery

   oblique intramural course of the vesiculo-ureteric junction.

8. There are several different types of renal calculus, depending on the chemical composition of the stone:

   calcium (oxalate or phosphate)

   struvite or 'triple phosphate' – usually secondary to urinary tract infections, e.g. *Proteus*

   uric acid – may be associated with gout

   cysteine

   xanthine

   other rare types.

9. Calcium stones represent approximately 75% of all nephrolithiases.

Question 38 – Answers

1. This is a kidney.

2. B – left renal vein

   C – left renal artery

   D – aorta

   E – inferior vena cava

   F – left ureter.

3. The left suprarenal (adrenal) gland.
4. From anterior to posterior: renal vein – renal artery (or arteries) – renal pelvis and ureter.
5. In this photograph the renal artery is passing in front of the renal vein. This is therefore the posterior aspect of the left kidney.
6. The kidneys lie in the paravertebral grooves at the levels of T12 to L3. The hilum is at the transpyloric plane (the left is slightly higher). They are retroperitoneal structures. Each kidney is surrounded by a renal capsule of fibrous tissue, i.e. within the perinephric fat. This fat is surrounded by the renal fascia (Gerota's fascia).
7. The posterior relations of the kidney (four muscles) are:
   - diaphragm (superiorly)
   - quadratus lumborum (inferiorly)
   - psoas major (medially)
   - transversus abdominis (laterally).
8. The kidneys are retroperitoneal.
9. The lymphatic drainage of the kidney is to the para-aortic nodes adjacent to the renal arteries. The upper pole may drain superiorly to the posterior mediastinal lymph nodes.
10. The dilated upper portion of the ureter is called the renal pelvis. This is formed by two or three major calyces, which are formed by the confluence of several minor calyces. Each minor calyx has a renal papilla draining into it, which is formed by the apices of several pyramids of renal medulla. The darker renal medulla is surrounded by the lighter-coloured renal cortex. The renal columns of cortex project inwards between the pyramids.
11. The functional unit of the kidney is the nephron. This comprises a glomerulus and a tubule system.
12. There are approximately 1 million nephrons per kidney.

Question 39 – Answers

1. This is an abdominal aortogram.
2. A – abdominal aorta
   B – right common iliac artery
   C – left common iliac artery
   D – left renal artery
   E – right renal artery
   F – splenic artery
   G – common hepatic artery
   H – superior mesenteric artery
   I – gastroduodenal artery
   J – left hepatic artery
   K – right hepatic artery
   L – inferior mesenteric artery.
3. The abdominal aorta starts in the midline as it passes through the diaphragm at the level of T12 (2.5 cm above the transpyloric plane). It runs in the

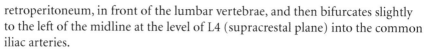

retroperitoneum, in front of the lumbar vertebrae, and then bifurcates slightly to the left of the midline at the level of L4 (supracrestal plane) into the common iliac arteries.

4. The midline branches are:

    coeliac axis (L1 upper)

    superior mesenteric artery (L1 lower)

    inferior mesenteric artery (L3).

    The paired branches are:

    inferior phrenic arteries (T12)

    suprarenal arteries (L1) – sometimes these arise from the renal arteries

    renal arteries (between L1 and L2)

    gonadal arteries (L2)

    four paired lumbar arteries (L1, L2, L3, L4).

5. An aneurysm is an abnormal dilation of an artery.

6. A true aneurysm contains all the layers of the vessel wall, whereas a false aneurysm does not. A false aneurysm is usually the result of trauma and leads to a fibrous capsule adjacent to and communicating with the lumen of the vessel but is not enclosed by the wall of that vessel.

7. The inferior vena cava has a longer course than the aorta as it forms at a lower level (L5) by the confluence of the common iliac veins, behind the right common iliac artery. It runs up in front of the lumbar vertebrae on the right of the aorta. It pierces the central tendon of the diaphragm at the level of T8 (higher than the aorta).

8. The portal vein is formed by the confluence of the superior mesenteric vein and the splenic vein. It lies in front of the inferior vena cava, behind the head of the pancreas and the first part of the duodenum. Other tributaries of the portal vein are the right and left gastric veins, the superior pancreaticoduodenal vein, the cystic vein and sometimes the periumbilical vein in the ligamentum teres (the remnant of the left umbilical vein). The portal vein ascends within the free edge of the lesser omentum (forming the anterior border of the foramen of Winslow), lying behind the bile duct and hepatic artery. At the porta hepatis it divides into right and left branches for the respective halves of the liver.

Question 40 – Answers

1. A – spermatic cord

    B – reflected aponeurosis of external oblique

    C – superficial inferior epigastric vein.

2. D – deep inguinal ring

    E – superficial inguinal ring.

3. This is the left inguinal region.

4. It is a cleft-like space, entirely between the layers of the abdominal wall. It is approximately 2 cm wide and runs above and parallel to the inguinal ligament. It extends from the deep ring (opening in the transversalis fascia) to the superficial ring (opening in the external oblique).

5. **anterior** – external oblique aponeurosis, reinforced laterally by internal oblique

   posterior – transversalis fascia, reinforced medially by conjoint tendon

   inferior – in-rolled edge of external oblique (i.e. inguinal ligament)

   superior – lower edge of internal oblique and transversus abdominis.

6. Running through the inguinal canal are the ilioinguinal nerve and in males the spermatic cord and in females the round ligament.

7. The mid-inguinal point is halfway between the anterior superior iliac spine and the pubic symphysis. This corresponds to the femoral artery pulse.

8. The midpoint of the inguinal ligament is halfway between the anterior superior iliac spine and the pubic tubercle. This corresponds to the deep inguinal ring. The mid-inguinal point is therefore medial to the midpoint of the inguinal ligament.

9. As the testes descend through the inguinal canal with the vas deferens and neurovascular structures, they take a contribution from the abdominal wall layers, which become fascial coverings. The layers of the scrotum and cord are:

   - skin of the scrotum derived from the abdominal skin
   - dartos muscle from abdominal Camper's fascia
   - dartos fascia from abdominal Scarpa's fascia
   - external spermatic fascia from external oblique muscle
   - cremaster muscle from internal oblique muscle
   - internal spermatic fascia from transversalis fascia
   - tunica vaginalis of the testes (and obliterated processus vaginalis of the cord) from the abdominal peritoneum.

   Note the transversus abdominis muscle does not contribute a layer to the cord or scrotum.

10. The contents of the spermatic cord are:

    - three arteries – testicular, cremasteric and artery of the vas deferens
    - three nerves – sympathetic, parasympathetic and genitofemoral nerve
    - three other structures – vas deferens, pampaniform plexus of veins and lymphatic vessels.

11. The testicular veins are formed by the merging pampaniform plexus of veins, which serve an important role in thermoregulation of the testes. The left testicular vein drains into the left renal vein. The right testicular vein drains directly into the inferior vena cava.

12. Because of the more oblique entry of the right testicular vein into the inferior vena cava, it is less likely to allow backflow of blood; varicoceles are therefore more common on the left side.

Question 41 – Answers

1. This is a CT scan of the abdomen at the level of L1 – the transpyloric plane.
2. A – right kidney
   B – left kidney
   C – liver
   D – stomach

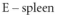

E – spleen
F – body of L1 vertebra
G – pancreas
H – aorta
I – left renal vein
J – inferior vena cava
K – superior mesenteric vein
L – right rectus abdominis muscle
M – second part of duodenum
N – right psoas major muscle
O – right quadratus lumborum muscle
P – superior mesenteric artery.

3. The transpyloric plane is halfway between the suprasternal notch and the superior pubic symphysis. At this level are the:
    termination of the spinal cord
    aorta gives off the superior mesenteric artery
    lateral border of the rectus abdominis muscle as it crosses the costal margin
    duodenojejunal junction
    L1 vertebra
    neck of the pancreas
    hila of the kidneys
    formation of the portal vein.

4. The stomach is a foregut structure and therefore is supplied by branches of the coeliac trunk. The lesser curve of the stomach is supplied by the right and left gastric arteries. The greater curve of the stomach is supplied by the right and left gastroepiploic arteries. The fundus is supplied by the short gastric arteries. The coeliac trunk divides into three branches – hepatic, splenic and left gastric arteries. The splenic artery gives off the short gastric and left gastroepiploic arteries. The hepatic artery gives off the right gastric and gastroduodenal arteries. The gastroduodenal artery divides into the superior pancreaticoduodenal and right gastroepiploic arteries.

5. The veins of the stomach correspond to the arteries. The lesser curve is drained by the right and left gastric veins. The greater curve is drained by the right and left gastroepiploic veins. The fundus is drained by the short gastric veins. The short gastric and left gastroepiploic veins drain into the splenic vein. The right gastroepiploic veins drain into the superior mesenteric vein. The right gastric vein drains directly into the portal vein. The portal vein is formed by the confluence of the superior mesenteric and splenic veins. Note the inferior mesenteric vein drains into the splenic vein.

6. The portosystemic anastomoses occur at the:
    oesophagus
    umbilicus
    rectum
    retroperitoneum.

7. The superior mesenteric artery provides the blood supply to the embryological midgut structures. The superior mesenteric artery arises from the abdominal aorta at the transpyloric plane (L1) behind the body of the pancreas. It then

passes anterior to the uncinate process of the pancreas and third part of the duodenum – that is, the pancreas and duodenum are wrapped around the superior mesenteric artery and vein. The branches are:
- inferior pancreaticoduodenal
- middle colic
- right colic
- several jejunal and ileal arteries
- ileocolic.

8. The duodenum is principally supplied by the superior and inferior pancreaticoduodenal arteries. The first 2 cm of the duodenum also receives blood from the hepatic, gastroduodenal, right gastric and right gastroepiploic arteries.

9. The pancreas is principally supplied by the splenic artery. The head of the pancreas is also supplied by the superior and inferior pancreaticoduodenal arteries.

10. The lumbar plexus is formed by the anterior rami of the L1–L5 spinal nerves. The plexus lies within the psoas major.

11. The nerves of the lumbar plexus are divided according to how they exit the psoas major muscle:
   - **Lateral:**
     - iliohypogastric nerve (L1)
     - ilioinguinal nerve (L1)
     - lateral cutaneous nerve of thigh (L2, L3)
     - femoral nerve (L2, L3, L4).
   - **Anterior:**
     - genitofemoral nerve (L1, L2).
   - **Medial:**
     - obturator nerve (L2, L3, L4)
     - lumbosacral trunk (L4, L5).

Question 42 – Answers

1. This is a double-contrast enema (barium and air).
   A – caecum
   B – appendix
   C – ascending colon
   D – transverse colon
   E – descending colon
   F – sigmoid colon
   G – rectum
   H – hepatic flexure
   I – splenic flexure.

2. The ascending colon, descending colon, hepatic and splenic flexures and rectum are all retroperitoneal.

3. The colon is a midgut structure from the ileocaecal junction to the splenic flexure and is supplied by the superior mesenteric artery. The remaining portion of the colon (splenic flexure to anus) is a hindgut structure and is

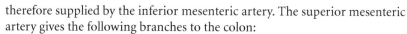

therefore supplied by the inferior mesenteric artery. The superior mesenteric artery gives the following branches to the colon:

- ileocolic
- right colic
- middle colic.

The inferior mesenteric artery gives the following branches to the colon:

- left colic
- several sigmoid arteries
- superior rectal.

These named arteries do not directly enter the colon but anastomose with each other to form the marginal artery (of Drummond) that runs alongside the colon, providing a collateral circulation.

4. The superior third of the rectum has peritoneum anteriorly and laterally. The middle third of the rectum has peritoneum anteriorly only. The lower third of the rectum has no peritoneum.

5. The following structures are **intraperitoneal**:

- stomach
- first part of the duodenum
- jejunum
- ileum
- transverse colon
- sigmoid colon
- tail of pancreas
- appendix
- caecum
- liver
- gallbladder
- uterus
- ovaries.

The following structures are **retroperitoneal**:

- kidneys
- ureters
- adrenal glands
- ascending and descending colon (including splenic and hepatic flexures)
- most of the pancreas (except the tip of the tail, which lies within the splenic peritoneum)
- second, third and fourth parts of duodenum
- inferior vena cava
- aorta
- lymph nodes around aorta
- bladder
- vagina.

6. The jejunum is darker red in colour, has a larger-calibre lumen, has a thicker wall, is more vascular, has longer vasa recta, has fewer arcades, has less fat in the mesentery and has deeper plicae circulares.

7. The large bowel has sacculations/haustrations, appendices epiploicae, tenia coli, a larger-calibre lumen and a thicker wall.

Question 43 – Answers

1. This is the inferior surface of the liver. The anterior surface is towards the top of the picture.
2. A – right lobe
    B – left lobe
    C – quadrate lobe
    D – caudate lobe.
3. E – gallbladder
    F – inferior vena cava
    G – falciform ligament
    H – ligamentum teres
    I – common bile duct
    J – portal vein
    K – hepatic artery.
4. Calot's triangle is formed by the cystic duct laterally, the common hepatic duct medially and the edge of the liver superiorly. It contains the right hepatic artery, the cystic artery and the right branch of the portal vein.
5. This is an opening between the greater sac (main peritoneal cavity) and the lesser sac (omental bursa).
6. **anterior** – free edge of the lesser omentum containing the portal triad
    posterior – inferior vena cava covered in peritoneum
    superior – caudate process of the liver
    inferior – first part of the duodenum covered in peritoneum.
7. This is Pringle's manoeuvre.
8. The portal triad are compressed between the finger and thumb as they run through the free edge of the lesser omentum: portal vein posteriorly, common bile duct on the right and hepatic artery on the left.
9. This manoeuvre can be used to temporarily stop the inflow of blood to the liver, e.g. to control haemorrhage from a liver laceration.
10. This is an endoscopic retrograde cholangiopancreatogram (ERCP).
11. A – ampulla of Vater
    B – pancreatic duct
    C – common bile duct
    D – fundus of gallbladder
    E – body of gallbladder
    F – neck of gallbladder
    G – cystic duct
    H – common hepatic duct
    I – left hepatic duct
    J – right hepatic duct.
12. The common bile duct enters the posteromedial wall of the second part of the duodenum at the ampulla of Vater.
13. The sphincter of Oddi regulates the flow of bile and is under neural and hormonal control.

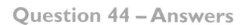

Question 44 – Answers

1. This is the inferior surface of the spleen.
2. The spleen lies on the left side of the upper abdomen. (This is a trick question to catch out the candidates thinking this organ is a kidney – easily done in the stress of the exam situation when handed a shrivelled up specimen!)
3. A – left kidney (renal impression)
   B – splenic flexure of colon (colonic impression)
   C – fundus/greater curve of stomach (gastric impression)
   D – tail of pancreas.
      Note the superoanterior surface usually has several notches to help you identify the gastric area.
4. The spleen is not normally palpable. It must at least double in size before its border is palpable under the costal margin.
5. The hepatorenal space (Morrison's pouch) is the most dependent area when supine. This is continuous with the right paracolic gutter and lies between the right kidney and the liver.
6. This is the most likely site for a collection of blood or pus to pool, leading to formation of an abscess.
7. The aponeuroses of three muscles make up the rectus sheath – external oblique, internal oblique and transversus abdominis. The rectus sheath has an anterior layer and a posterior layer. The superior three-quarters is different from the inferior quarter. The arcuate line demarcates the boundary between the two regions and lies 3 cm below the umbilicus. Superiorly, the anterior layer is made up of the aponeurosis of external oblique and half of the internal oblique muscles. The posterior layer is made up of the aponeurosis of the other half of the internal oblique and the transversus abdominis muscles. Inferiorly, all three muscle layers pass anteriorly. There is no posterior layer of sheath. The rectus abdominis muscle is in direct contact with the transversalis fascia.
8.   skin
   subcutaneous fat
   Scarpa's fascia
   linea alba
   transversalis fascia
   extraperitoneal fat
   peritoneum.

Question 45 – Answers

1. This is a female pelvis.
2. A – symphysis pubis
   B – bladder
   C – uterus
   D – rectum
   E – urethra
   F – vagina

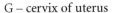

G – cervix of uterus

H – recto-uterine pouch (of Douglas)

I – anal canal

J – sigmoid colon

K – body of L5 vertebra

L – body of S1 vertebra

M – cauda equina.

3. This is the pelvic inlet.

4. The urethra starts at the bladder neck as the pre-prostatic urethra, descends through the prostate gland as the prostatic urethra, and exits the prostate gland to become the membranous urethra, which then enters the bulb of the penis to become the spongy urethra. The spongy urethra passes through the penis to end as the external urethral meatus.

5. The membranous urethra is surrounded by the external urethral sphincter. This muscle relaxes during the voiding of urine.

6. The prostatic urethra is the most dilatable.

7. The membranous urethra is the least dilatable part of the urethra.

8. This cystoscopy is from a male patient.

9. A – external urethral orifice

   B – penile urethra mucosa

   C – intrabulbar fossa

   D – opening to membranous urethra

   E – membranous urethra mucosa

   F – verumontanum (seminal colliculus)

   G – urethral crest

   H – opening of prostatic utricle

   I – prostatic sinus

   J – internal urethral orifice.

10. The prostatic utricle is a small blind-ending sac, a vestigial structure that is the homologue of the uterus. On either side of this (not seen in the photography) is the slit-like opening of the ejaculatory ducts.

11. The prostatic ducts open into the prostatic sinuses on either side of the urethral crest.

Question 46 – Answers

1. This is the right hip bone (or innominate bone).

2. A – anterior superior iliac spine

   B – iliac crest

   C – anterior inferior iliac spine

   D – obturator foramen

   E – greater sciatic notch

   F – ischial spine

   G – ischial tuberosity

   H – pubic tubercle

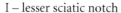

     I – lesser sciatic notch

     J – iliac fossa

     K – arcuate line

     L – superior ramus of pubis

     M – inferior ramus of pubis

     N – iliac tuberosity.

3. X – ischium

     Y – pubis

     Z – ilium.

4. The ilium, ischium and pubis meet in the acetabulum (meaning 'vinegar cup') to form a 'Mercedes' symbol.

5. The inguinal ligament attaches between the anterior superior iliac spine and the pubic tubercle.

6. O and P are the articular surfaces of the hip bone. O is the articular surface for the sacroiliac joint. This area is covered with hyaline cartilage. It is a synovial joint (the strongest in the body). P is the articular surface for the pubic symphysis. This area is covered by a thin layer of hyaline cartilage, which attaches to the opposite side through a thick fibrocartilaginous disc. This is a secondary cartilaginous joint.

7. Iliacus originates from the hollow of the iliac fossa, passes beneath the inguinal ligament and inserts into the psoas tendon.

Question 47

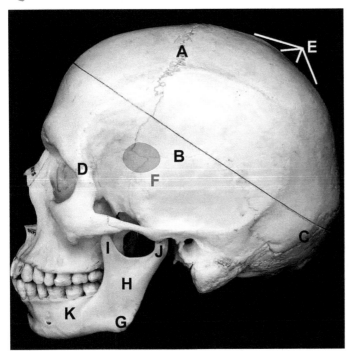

1. What are the names of the sutures labelled A–E?
2. What is the name of the most superior region of the cranium?
3. What is the red-shaded area labelled F?
4. What four bones articulate at this area?
5. What structure runs behind this area?
6. What is the clinical significance of this area?
7. Identify the parts of the mandible labelled G–K.
8. What are the layers of the scalp?
9. Are there any areas of the cranium that are not covered with periosteum? If so, where?
10. Describe the type of ossification that occurs in the fetal cranium and the fetal mandible.

Question 48

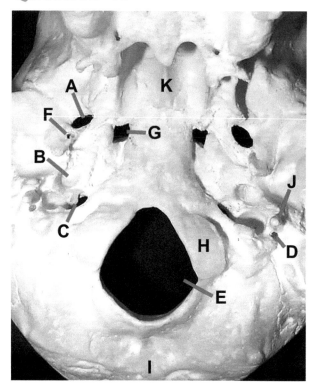

1. Identify the foramina labelled A–G. What structures pass through each one?
2. Identify the points labelled H–K.
3. With how many bones does the sphenoid articulate? What are they?
4. How many cranial nerves are there? What are their names?
5. What are the divisions of the fifth cranial nerve?
6. Describe the sensory distribution of the divisions of the fifth cranial nerve.
7. What are the muscles supplied by the fifth cranial nerve?
8. The mandibular division of the trigeminal nerve (V3) divides into 'cat of nine tails'. Describe these branches.
9. What structures pass through foramen ovale?
10. How could you clinically differentiate between an upper motor neuron lesion and a lower motor neuron lesion of the facial (seventh cranial) nerve?

Question 49

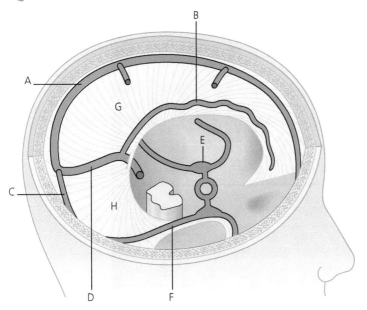

1. Identify the points labelled A–H.
2. What are the venous sinuses?
3. Describe the arrangement of the venous drainage of the brain.
4. What are the emissary veins?
5. What is the cavernous sinus? Describe its anatomy.
6. Which structures pass through the cavernous sinus?
7. Describe the clinical relevance of the cavernous sinus.
8. What is the source of cerebrospinal fluid (CSF)?
9. Describe the complete course of the CSF from the lateral ventricle.
10. What is the clinical condition associated with obstruction of the flow of CSF?

Question 50

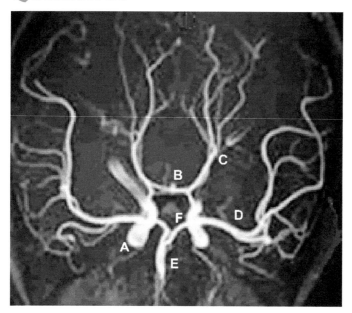

1. Identify the vessels labelled A–F.
2. What is the name of this anastomosis of vessels?
3. Describe the course of the internal carotid artery.
4. What are the three major intracranial branches of the internal carotid artery?
5. What are the two terminal branches of the internal carotid artery? Which of these is the larger vessel?
6. Which vessels merge to form the basilar artery?
7. What structures are supplied by the basilar artery?
8. What are the terminal divisions of the basilar artery?
9. Give the definition of a berry aneurysm.
10. Briefly describe the pathophysiological process that leads to the formation of a berry aneurysm.
11. What is the clinical significance of a berry aneurysm?

Question 51

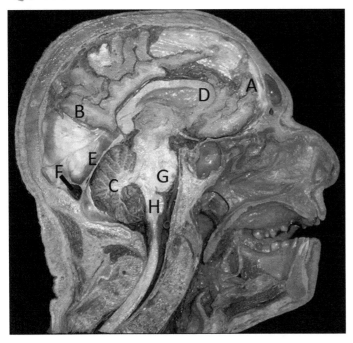

1. Identify the parts labelled A–H.
2. What are gyri and sulci?
3. What separates the temporal lobe from the frontal and parietal lobes?
4. Which structure links the two main cerebral hemispheres?
5. Within the cerebral cortex, which regions are involved in sensory information and motor signals?
6. What is the location of the visual cortex?
7. What is the histological composition of the cerebrum?
8. What is Broca's area? Describe its topographical location.
9. What is Wernicke's area? Describe its topographical location.
10. What is the clinical significance of these areas?

Question 52

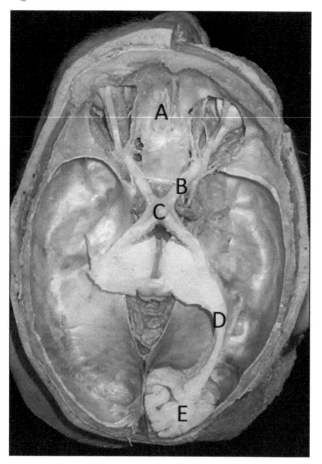

1. Identify the structures labelled A–E.
2. Which cranial nerves carry parasympathetic fibres?
3. Which structures accompany the optic (second cranial) nerve through its passage in the optic canal?
4. In which structure does the optic tract terminate?
5. What visual deficit results from a lesion at the central optic chiasm?
6. What are the divisions of the oculomotor (third cranial) nerve? What structures do they innervate?
7. Describe the pathophysiological process involved in brain swelling causing oculomotor (third cranial) nerve dysfunction.
8. Describe the anatomy of the trochlear (fourth cranial) nerve.
9. What structure is innervated by the abducens (sixth cranial) nerve?
10. What clinical deficit results from a trochlear (fourth cranial) nerve lesion?

Question 53

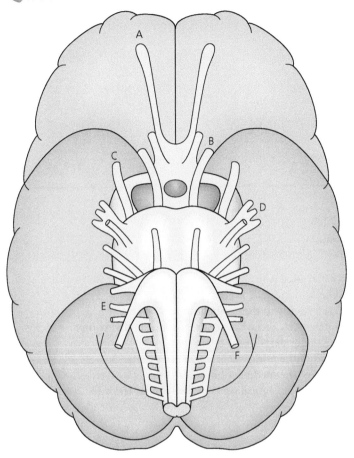

1. Identify the structures A–F.
2. Describe the origin of the vestibulocochlear (eighth cranial) nerve.
3. Through which structure does the vestibulocochlear (eighth cranial) nerve leave the posterior cranial fossa?
4. What structure has parasympathetic innervation via the glossopharyngeal (ninth cranial) nerve?
5. Briefly describe the clinical examination of the trigeminal (fifth cranial) nerve.
6. What is the function of the abducens (sixth cranial) nerve, and how might you clinically test it?
7. What are the seven major branches of the vagus (tenth cranial) nerve?
8. How might you clinically examine the vagus (tenth cranial) nerve?

Question 54

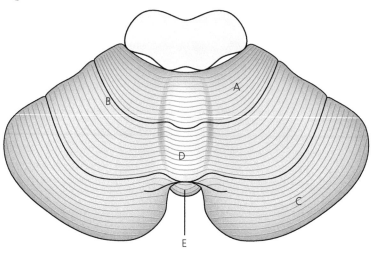

1. Identify the points labelled A–E.
2. Where is the cerebellum located? What is its main role?
3. Describe the arterial supply to the cerebellum.
4. What are the basal ganglia, and what are the five nuclei that comprise them?
5. What are the three major parts of the brain stem?
6. What is the function of the pons?
7. What is the function of the medulla oblongata?
8. What are the characteristic clinical signs of a cerebellar lesion?

Question 55

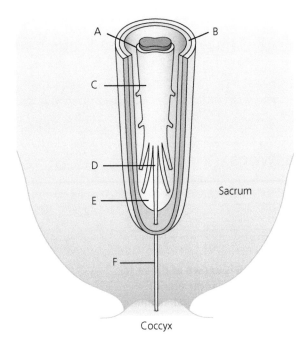

1. What are the three meningeal layers?
2. What separates the dura mater from the arachnoid mater?
3. Identify the points labelled A–F.
4. What are the ascending spinal pathways, and what are their functions?
5. What are the descending spinal pathways, and what are their functions?
6. In anatomical terms, what causes extradural (epidural) and subdural haemorrhages?
7. How could you differentiate between an extradural and a subdural haematoma on a computed tomography (CT) scan of the head?
8. What is spina bifida?

Question 47 – Answers

1. A – coronal suture
    B – squamous suture
    C – lamboid suture
    D – zygomaticofrontal suture
    E – sagittal suture.
2. The most superior region of the skull is known as the vertex.
3. The red-shaded area labelled F is known as the pterion.
4. The pterion is the junction of the frontal, parietal, temporal and sphenoid bones.
5. The anterior branch of the middle meningeal artery runs behind the pterion.
6. The pterion is a weak point of the skull and may be fractured by a blow to the temporal region (e.g. from a cricket ball). A fracture may lacerate the middle meningeal artery, leading to an extradural haematoma.
7. G – angle
    H – ramus
    I – coronoid process
    J – head
    K – body.
8. The layers of the scalp are (from superficial to deep) (remember 'SCALP'):
    skin
    connective tissue (containing vessels and nerves)
    aponeurosis of occipitalis/frontalis muscles (galea)
    loose connective (areolar) tissue
    pericranium (periosteum).
9. The temporal fossae of the lateral skull are not covered with periosteum. This is the point of attachment of the temporalis muscles. The periosteum around this fossa is continuous with the deep temporal fascia over the top of this muscle.
10. The flat bones of the skull vault, the face and the mandible all undergo intramembranous ossification, whereas the bones of the skull base undergo endochondral ossification.

Question 48 – Answers

1. A – foramen ovale
    - mandibular division of the trigeminal nerve
    B – carotid canal
    - internal carotid artery
    - sympathetic plexus
    C – jugular foramen
    - internal jugular vein (formed by inferior petrosal and sigmoid sinuses)
    - glossopharyngeal nerve
    - vagus nerve
    - accessory nerve
    D – stylomastoid foramen
    - facial nerve
    - stylomastoid artery
    E – foramen magnum
    - medulla and surrounding meninges
    - spinal roots of accessory nerve
    - anterior and posterior spinal and vertebral arteries
    F – foramen spinosum
    - middle meningeal vessels
    G – foramen lacerum
    - internal carotid artery (passes into foramen lacerum from carotid canal).
2. H – occipital condyle
    I – external occipital protuberance
    J – styloid process
    K – vomer.
3. The sphenoid articulates with eight other bones:
    - temporal
    - parietal
    - frontal
    - vomer
    - occipital
    - zygomatic
    - palatine
    - ethmoidal.
4. There are 12 cranial nerves:
    I – olfactory
    II – optic
    III – oculomotor
    IV – trochlea
    V – trigeminal
    VI – abducens
    VII – facial
    VIII – vestibulocochlear
    IX – glossopharyngeal

X – vagus
XI – accessory
XII – hypoglossal.

5. The fifth cranial or trigeminal nerve supplies sensation to the face and motor supply to the muscles of mastication. The divisions are:
   - ophthalmic
   - maxillary
   - mandibular.

6. The **ophthalmic division** supplies sensation to the forehead, upper eyelids, eye, anterior nose and nasal mucosa. The **maxillary division** supplies sensation to the cheek, lower eyelid, lateral nose, upper teeth, upper lip and maxillary sinuses. The **mandibular division** supplies sensation to the skin over the mandible, lower teeth and lip, temporal skin, and lower oral cavity.

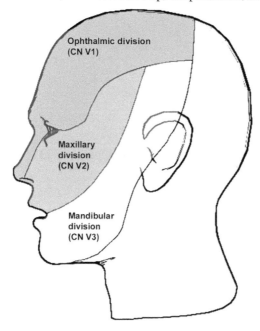

7. The muscles supplied by the trigeminal (fifth cranial) nerve are:
   - muscles of mastication (medial and lateral pterygoids, masseter and temporalis muscles)
   - tensor tympani
   - mylohyoid
   - anterior belly of digastric muscle.

8. After passing through the foramen ovale into the infratemporal fossa, the mandibular division of the trigeminal nerve divides into multiple branches. These consist of an anterior group, which are all motor except one, and a posterior group, which are all sensory except one.
   - **Anterior group:**
     – two branches to lateral pterygoid
     – two branches to temporalis

    – nerve to masseter

    – buccal nerve (only sensory branch).

  Posterior group:

    – auriculotemporal nerve

    – lingual nerve

    – inferior alveolar nerve (gives off nerve to myelohyoid – only motor branch).

9. The structures passing through foramen ovale can be remembered using the mnemonic 'OVALE':

  otic ganglion

  V3 (mandibular or third division of cranial nerve V)

  accessory meningeal artery

  lesser petrosal nerve

  emissary veins.

10. The superior facial muscles have bilateral innervations from both the right and left sides of the motor cortex. Upper motor neuron lesions therefore usually have sparing of ipsilateral superior facial muscle function. A lower motor neuron lesion, however, will result in complete ipsilateral facial paralysis (superior and inferior).

Question 49 – Answers

1. A – superior sagittal sinus

  B – inferior sagittal sinus

  C – transverse sinus

  D – straight sinus

  E – cavernous sinus

  F – sigmoid sinus

  G – falx cerebri

  H – tentorium cerebelli.

2. The venous sinuses are channels within the dura mater that direct venous blood and cerebrospinal fluid (CSF) from the brain to the systemic venous circulation, and contain no valves.

3. A network of cerebral veins drains into the venous sinuses:

  superior sagittal sinus – lies in the superior falx cerebri and runs from the crista gali anteriorly to the internal occipital protuberance posteriorly (confluence of sinuses)

  inferior sagittal sinus – lies in the inferior border of the falx cerebri and joins the great cerebral vein to become the straight sinus

  straight sinus – formed by the confluence of the inferior sagittal sinus and the great cerebral vein and runs inferoposteriorly to the internal occipital protuberance (confluence of sinuses)

  transverse sinuses – (right and left) pass laterally from the internal occipital protuberance (confluence of sinuses) to become the sigmoid sinuses

  sigmoid sinuses – curve medially and then exit through the jugular foramina to become the internal jugular veins

occipital sinus – runs superiorly from the epidural plexus of veins to the confluence of sinuses

cavernous sinuses – lie on either side of the sella turcica; these sinuses drain the ophthalmic, sphenoparietal and middle cerebral veins into the superior and inferior petrosal sinuses

superior petrosal sinuses – run from the cavernous sinuses to the junction of the transverse and sigmoid sinuses

inferior petrosal sinuses – run from the cavernous sinuses to empty directly into the internal jugular veins

basilar sinuses – connect the inferior petrosal sinuses with the epidural plexus of veins.

4. The emissary veins connect the intracranial and extracranial veins.

5. The cavernous sinuses are paired venous sinuses about 2 cm long on either side of the sella turcica and lateral to the sphenoid air sinuses, immediately posterior to the optic chiasm. Draining into these sinuses are the superior and inferior ophthalmic veins, the superficial middle cerebral vein and the sphenoparietal sinuses. The cavernous sinuses communicate with each other via the intercavernous sinuses and drain into the inferior and superior petrosal sinuses.

6. The cavernous sinuses contain the internal carotid artery, the oculomotor (third cranial) nerve, the trochlear (fourth cranial) nerve, the ophthalmic and maxillary divisions of the trigeminal (fifth cranial) nerve, the abducens (sixth cranial) nerve and the sympathetic plexus.

7. Infections or tumours of the face may spread through the facial veins and ophthalmic veins (valveless) into the cavernous sinuses, causing thrombosis. This condition manifests as a swollen, painful, venous congested ipsilateral eye, progressive loss of vision and the development of third, fourth, fifth and sixth cranial nerve palsies. The condition may also spread quickly to the contralateral sinus.

8. CSF is formed by the choroid plexus in the cerebral ventricles.

9. From the lateral ventricle, CSF flows to the interventricular foramen (of Monro), into the third ventricle, and through the cerebral aqueduct (of Sylvius), draining into the fourth ventricle. From the fourth ventricle, CSF passes through the foramen of Magendie (medial) and the foramina of Luschka (lateral) into the cisterns in the subarachnoid space.

10. Obstruction in the flow or uptake of CSF will result in dilation of the ventricles and raised intracranial pressure. This is known as hydrocephalus.

Question 50 – Answers

1. A – internal carotid artery
   B – anterior communicating artery
   C – anterior cerebral artery
   D – middle cerebral artery
   E – basilar artery
   F – posterior communicating artery.
2. This anastomosis is known as the circle of Willis.

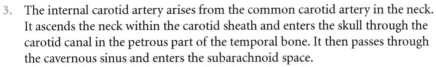

3. The internal carotid artery arises from the common carotid artery in the neck. It ascends the neck within the carotid sheath and enters the skull through the carotid canal in the petrous part of the temporal bone. It then passes through the cavernous sinus and enters the subarachnoid space.
4. The major intracranial branches of the internal carotid artery are:
    - ophthalmic artery
    - posterior communicating artery
    - anterior choroid artery.
5. The terminal vessels of the internal carotid artery are the middle cerebral and anterior cerebral arteries. The middle cerebral artery is the larger of the two.
6. The basilar artery is formed from the two joining vertebral arteries on the surface of the pons.
7. The cerebellum and the pons are supplied by the basilar artery.
8. The basilar artery gives off four major branches:
    - pontine branch
    - anterior inferior cerebellar artery
    - labyrinthine artery
    - superior cerebellar artery.
    It then terminates by dividing into the left and right posterior cerebral arteries.
9. A berry aneurysm (saccular aneurysm) is a sac-like out-pouching in the wall of a cerebral blood vessel that sometimes appears berry-shaped.
10. Berry aneurysms are congenital malformations and result from an inherent weakness and thinning in the vessel wall. Specifically, there is usually a lack of tunica media and elastic lamina around the dilated part. These areas are susceptible to increased hydrostatic pressure from systemic hypertension and subsequently bulge out.
11. A berry aneurysm may spontaneously rupture due to its weakness and lead to a subarachnoid haemorrhage. It may also cause symptoms by enlarging and compressing neighbouring structures.

Question 51 – Answers

1. A – frontal lobe
   B – calcarine sulcus (fissure)
   C – cerebellum
   D – corpus callosum
   E – tentorium cerebella
   F – transverse sinus
   G – pons
   H – medulla.
2. Gyri are elevated folds on the cerebral hemisphere, and sulci are the grooves between them. This structural pattern serves to increase the surface area of the cerebrum.
3. The lateral sulcus (Sylvian fissure) separates the temporal lobe from the frontal and parietal lobes.

4. The corpus callosum is the white matter structure that links the two main cerebral hemispheres.
5. In the cerebral cortex, the **postcentral gyrus** (the gyrus of the parietal lobe immediately posterior to the central sulcus) is involved in conducting sensory information. The **precentral gyrus** (the gyrus of the frontal lobe immediately anterior to the central sulcus) is involved in relaying motor signals.
6. The visual cortex is located in the occipital lobe.
7. The cerebral cortex is divided broadly into two main histological subtypes – the grey matter (which is superficial) and the white matter (which is deep). Grey matter is largely composed of neuronal cell bodies, whereas the white matter is formed by the axonal tracts of neurons.
8. There are two distinct areas within the brain that are responsible for speech. Broca's area is one of these; it is located in the left inferior frontal gyrus (Brodman areas 44 and 45). It is named after the French pathologist Pierre Broca.
9. Wernicke's area is the other region that contributes to speech function. It is located in the left posterior part of the superior temporal gyrus (Brodman area 22). It is named after the German neurologist Carl Wernicke.
10. Any lesions within Broca's area result in expressive aphasia, while lesions within Wernicke's area are associated with receptive aphasia.

Question 52 – Answers

1. A – olfactory (first cranial) nerve filaments (passing through cribriform plate)
   B – optic (second cranial) nerve
   C – optic chiasm
   D – optic tract
   E – occipital (visual) cortex.
2. The oculomotor (third cranial), facial (seventh cranial), glossopharyngeal (ninth cranial) and vagus (tenth cranial) nerves carry parasympathetic fibres.
3. The ophthalmic artery and central retinal vein accompany the optic (second cranial) nerve through its passage in the optic canal.
4. The optic tract terminates in the lateral geniculate body of the thalamus and the visual cortex in the occipital lobe.
5. A lesion at the optic chiasm (such as a pituitary tumour) will cause impingement on decussating fibres from both right and left optic nerves. There is a resultant loss of vision in the temporal (lateral) visual field of both eyes. This is known as bitemporal hemianopia.
6. The oculomotor (third cranial) nerve has superior and inferior divisions. The **superior division** supplies superior rectus and levator palpebrae superioris muscles. The **inferior division** supplies inferior and medial rectus, inferior oblique, and the ciliary and sphincter pupillae muscles.
7. Brain swelling may cause an increase in intracranial pressure, eventually leading to uncal herniation and subsequent compression of the oculomotor (third cranial) nerve. This causes the characteristic clinical sign of a fixed

(unresponsive) and dilated pupil on the ipsilateral side to the herniation, due to a loss of parasympathetic innervation to the sphincter pupillae muscle.

8. The trochlear (fourth cranial) nerve emerges from the posterior midbrain and runs anteriorly beneath the free edge of the tentorium cerebella. It then passes under the oculomotor (third cranial) nerve to pierce the dura mater of the lateral wall of the cavernous sinus. From here, the nerve passes into the orbit via the superior orbital fissure and finally travels medially into the superior oblique.

9. The abducens (sixth cranial) nerve innervates the lateral rectus muscle. (Remember the formula $LR_6(SO_4)3$ to denote the innervations of the extraocular muscles – lateral rectus by sixth cranial nerve, superior oblique by the fourth cranial nerve, and all others by the third cranial nerve.)

10. Lesions of the trochlear (fourth cranial) nerve result in a failure to depress the eye, most noticeable during adduction.

Question 53 – Answers

1. A – olfactory (first cranial) nerve
   B – oculomotor (third cranial) nerve
   C – trochlear (fourth cranial) nerve
   D – trigeminal (fifth cranial) nerve
   E – vagus (tenth cranial) nerve
   F – hypoglossal (twelfth cranial) nerve.

2. The vestibulocochlear (eighth cranial) nerve has separate vestibular and cochlear branches arising at a groove between the pons and medulla.

3. The vestibulocochlear (eighth cranial) nerve leaves the posterior cranial fossa through the internal acoustic meatus, in the petrous part of the temporal bone.

4. The parotid gland has parasympathetic innervation from the glossopharyngeal (ninth cranial) nerve. Note that the facial (seventh cranial) nerve passes through the substance of the gland but does not innervate it.

5. Rapid assessment of the function of the trigeminal (fifth cranial) nerve may be performed by testing the sensation of the face (sensory function) and palpating the masseter and temporalis muscles as the patient bites down (motor function).

6. The abducens (sixth cranial) nerve provides motor innervations to the lateral rectus muscle of the eye. It may be clinically tested by observing extraocular movements in the patient, particularly abduction of both eyes.

7. The seven major branches of the vagus (tenth cranial) nerve are as follows:
   - **meningeal branch** – gives sensation to the dura mater in the posterior cranial fossa
   - **auricular branch** – gives sensation to the posterior aspect of the ear
   - **superior laryngeal branch** – the external laryngeal branch supplies motor innervation to the inferior constrictor and cricothyroid muscles, and the internal laryngeal branch gives sensation to the superior larynx

      recurrent laryngeal branch – gives sensation to the inferior larynx and supplies motor innervation to all laryngeal intrinsic muscles except the cricothyroid

      nerve to carotid body and sinus

      motor branch to pharyngeal plexus

      parasympathetic branches to thoracic and abdominal visceral structures.

8. The function of the vagus (tenth cranial) nerve may be tested by asking the patient to phonate with an open mouth (say 'ah') and observing midline elevation of the soft palate and uvula.

Question 54 – Answers

1. A – anterior lobe

   B – primary fissure

   C – posterior lobe

   D – vermis

   E – vallecula.

2. The cerebellum is located in the posterior cranial fossa. It has a complex role in the coordination of movement and posture.

3. There are three arteries that supply the cerebellum:

   superior cerebellar artery – branch of the basilar artery

   anterior inferior cerebellar artery – branch of the basilar artery

   posterior inferior cerebellar artery – branch of the vertebral artery.

4. The basal ganglia are grey matter nuclei located in the base of the cerebral hemispheres. They are involved in coordination of voluntary motor function. The five nuclei that comprise the basal ganglia are:

   caudate nucleus

   putamen

   globus pallidus

   substantia nigra

   subthalamic nucleus.

5. The three major parts of the brain stem are the midbrain (mesencephalon), pons and medulla oblongata.

6. The pons regulates hearing and balance and contains various autonomic centres.

7. The medulla oblongata contains tracts passing to and from the spinal cord, and contains autonomic centres that regulate cardiorespiratory and gastrointestinal physiological mechanisms.

8. The classic clinical signs attributed to cerebellar lesions can be denoted by the mnemonic 'DANISH':

   dysdiadochokinesis

   ataxia

   nystagmus

   intention tremor

   staccato speech

   hypotonia (global).

Question 55 – Answers

1. The three meningeal layers are, from superficial to deep:
    - dura mater
    - arachnoid mater
    - pia mater.
2. The dura mater is separated from the arachnoid mater by the subdural space (a potential space).
3. A schematic representation of the distal spinal cord:
    A – pia mater
    B – arachnoid mater
    C – conus medullaris
    D – cauda equina
    E – lumbar cistern
    F – filum terminale.
4. The ascending spinal pathways are somatic sensory neural pathways that travel cranially along the spinal cord. They are the **posterior-column medial lemniscus** (or **dorsal**) tract and **spinothalamic** tract. The dorsal tract conveys light touch, vibration and joint-position sense (proprioception). The spinothalamic tract conducts pain and temperature sensation.
5. The descending spinal pathways are motor neural pathways that travel caudally along the spinal cord. They are the **corticospinal** (or **pyramidal**) tract and the **reticulospinal** tract. These pathways conduct motor nerve fibres to the musculature.
6. An **extradural haemorrhage** (within the potential space between the dura mater and the skull) is caused by rupture of an artery (e.g. middle meningeal artery). A **subdural haemorrhage** is caused by rupture of the cerebral veins as they travel from the cerebrum through to the venous sinuses.
7. On both axial and coronal views of a CT scan, an extradural haematoma will have a lenticular (lens-like) appearance, whereas a subdural haematoma usually has a crescent-like appearance.
8. Spina bifida refers to a group of congenital malformations that result from the failure of fusion of the two halves of the neural arches, most commonly found in the lumbosacral region. Spina bifida occulta is usually without symptoms or consequence. Spina bifida cystic permits protrusion of a meningeal cyst, either with no neural content (meningocoele) or with spinal cord or cauda equine contained (myelomeningocoele). A myelomeningocoele often results in lower-limb paralysis and bowel or bladder dysfunction.

T - #0862 - 101024 - C138 - 234/156/6 - PB - 9781444170191 - Gloss Lamination